Neuroleptic Malignant Syndrome

Deadly Drugging of Dementia

Victoria Allen

ISBN: 978-1-8383758-0-5 (paperback)
ISBN: 978-1-8383758-1-2 (ebook)

Preface

The Isle of Man is a beautiful windswept small island, set between the U.K. and Ireland in the Irish Sea. It has a small population of under 85,000 and can be very insular. It has its own parliament called Tynwald, along with separate legislation and laws. It is a "crown dependency".

This book is set in the Isle of Man amongst the "goings-on", of the small island hospital. The book takes readers through some closely guarded secrets and exposes the reality of the blundering process when things go wrong; very wrong. Close relationships, acquaintances, " boys' clubs", within the hierarchy of both government and hospital management, protectively stick together in a desperate attempt to keep truths hidden. Mental Health Services flounder to protect themselves and the Government, amid neglect and scandal. The book aims to explore the question of whether psychiatry is playing a dangerous role in trying to defend their drug-peddling careers, whilst Government covers them too.

The book exposes corruption and deceit riddled through the ranks and provides truth-based facts, to enable the reader to draw their own conclusions.

Some medical reference and aspects to the book may prove intense reading, and therefore, I invite the lay-reader to skip these areas if required.

It begs the question, have we gone from obvious, physically straight-jacketing patients, to less-obvious, but dangerous levels of chemically straight-jacketing them instead?

More importantly, has anything now changed on the island and can a problem be solved in the very environment in which it was created?

In memory of my beautiful cousin, Jeanette Hector;
An amazing lady with a true gift for laughter.

*"Assumption is the Mother of all F***k-ups".*
Somebody, somewhere once said.

1

The Dawning

I had gently woken up that morning, taking more than half an hour to rouse from the sumptuously comfortable bed. I had lain awake savouring the sweet trill songs from the birds outside. How tremendous to be truly alive again with time to enjoy the exquisitely beautiful, yet simple things that life had to offer. It was just over one week since our last guest had left, meaning an end to the dreaded 6.30 am alarm, excitedly beeping to wake me and entice me out of bed. The picturesque country house that we owned in the Isle of Man, could only accommodate six people at any given time, but with myself and my husband, Nigel, running it alone, the work and hours could be very tiring. We loved doing it and meeting so many interesting people, but it was exhausting at times, so after six months of hard work, it was time for a well-earned rest; to have our delightful house back to ourselves. Enjoy the serenity of the glen setting; the greenery of the trees; the gurgling stream at the bottom of the garden along with all of the busy birds that visited.

The sky was clear blue and the day sunny. I was suddenly blissfully aware of my new-found freedom again. Shani, the recently adopted silver Bengal cat, stretched her paws out in front and gave a huge yawn, before rubbing her head on my face; leaving tickly little hairs behind. I told her how pretty she was before she elegantly jumped off the bed and trotted off for her breakfast. Such a perfect start to the day. So lucky.

The kettle boiled and the coffee was promptly made. We strolled off into the garden with it, to enjoy the "guest experience". The grass was glistening with the wet dew on each blade. The lawn was immaculately green and complimented the property perfectly. Our Victorian-style house was quaint and cosy-looking with natural bare Manx-stone walls that added to the character of the guesthouse. The morning air was cool and refreshing, with a damp, earthy leaf smell. The whole house and plot were surrounded by a variety of trees, with so many shades of green adding to the backdrop. The house was snuggled at the base of a valley. Birds were flitting between trees; the still, quiet morning broken only by sweet bird song and honeybees hovering from flower to flower. They were humming peacefully around the tranquil glen, providing a delicate accompaniment for the birdsong. I heaved in a deep long breath, with a subconscious, "thank you", as I angled my eyes towards the sky. We sat on the wooden garden swing. Shani waited for me to settle, then jumped up onto my lap. One hand was holding my cup and the other was stroking her; she purred blissfully with appreciation, gazing at me with her huge beautiful green eyes. Eyes that were so large that she appeared owl-like. Such a pretty girl, I reminded her. Birds were flying swiftly passed us, en-route to the honeysuckle that climbed over the trellised walkway. There were mainly Blue Tits; Great Tits and Coal Tits. All enjoying the bright red honeysuckle berries. Shani would never bother with the birds, unless they were pecking on the lawn. She would then crouch with her belly dragging along the grass, stalking them. Then she would charge at them with her full force. Yet she was never quite adept enough as they flew off, before tormenting her by returning only minutes later. I heaved in another big sigh. A sigh of perfection. I wanted to stay there forever, sitting on the swing drinking coffee (or wine), just as we were, but with the guest-free solitude, came the chores of washing, cleaning and renewing the décor, for next season.

We all returned to the house across the dew-kissed lawn; the cat chasing butterflies and flies as we went. I enjoyed seeing her humour back after being such a sad little thing, not so long ago.

Back at the house, I popped my coffee cup in the kitchen – a lovely dark wood country-style kitchen with glossy cream and burgundy tiles, which was a little shady during the day, but beautifully lit and cosy in the evening. Handmade kitchen units and an unusual floor to ceiling, separating room divider, between the kitchen and dining area, added to the quaintness of the oak beamed ceiling. Part of my usual routine was to check the answer-phone machine after being out in the garden. I went into our private lounge; a superbly light room; cosy but bright with two windows exposing the true beauty of the glen setting and the trees. We had stowed-away our super-comfy sofa bed that we slept on during the tourist season. The room was perfectly in order today. The answerphone was flashing and showed there was one new message. Another booking no doubt. I pressed the play button and listened; pen in hand, ready to write the potential client's telephone number down. As I was listening to the voice talking, the hairs on the back of my neck raised and a shudder rippled down my back. My blood turned cold. It was my father, Jim's voice, but not as I recognised it.

The message finished. I had heard nothing of the content and noticed only the short staccato, but slow manner, in which my father spoke. I replayed the message. He explained that he had woken-up but did not "feel right". He was exhausted and tired and was unable to walk normally. His coordination had gone. His speech was slurred and slow. He had rang the Day Care Centre where my father took my mother, Judith, twice a week, who had dementia. He had explained how he felt to the senior care worker there and she had suggested that he had suffered a possible stroke, and she had urged him to ring his doctors' surgery. He rang the surgery and explained everything to the receptionist. She gave him an appointment, for just after lunchtime. I couldn't contain my shock when I returned his call. "For God's sake", I told him, "You need an ambulance, or a home visit, not an appointment". This riled my father. He informed me that he had relayed all of this to the surgery and had been given an appointment. They were very busy and I was not to make a fuss. I relented on this and told him that I would drive over to see him at his house and take him to the appointment. I promptly collected my handbag and shouted to Nigel and relayed the scenario to him. He was equally perturbed and after collecting our things together and locking the house, we both hurried and set-off in the car.

While driving the ten miles or so over the mountain to Ramsey, my stomach was heavy; sick to the pit. My throat and neck felt enlarged with a heavy beating lump lower down in my chest. I was worried sick. My mother, Judith, had recently been diagnosed with suspected Alzheimer's dementia. She had a CT scan some months earlier, showing no apparent signs of the disease, but it was still a suspected diagnosis. Her behaviour and personality had certainly changed in recent months. She had most noticeably started to wear bizarre clothing; odd socks; cowboy hats; odd shoes; make-up applied in a child-like manner. She had needed direction to the bathroom in our house now, despite the fact that we had lived in the house for nearly nine years. It appeared as if she was almost in a permanent state of drunkenness. Her walk was slower and her feet dragged slightly. They were swollen too, like fat, chubby baby feet. She was a very young looking, attractive, sixty nine year old lady, with high cheek bones and arched eyebrows framing her piercing green eyes. Her hair was dark chocolate brown, but more recently coloured a deep auburn colour. A very feminine, and eloquent lady, with broad shoulders and an athletic build. She was often mistaken for my father's daughter – she would laugh at this, slightly embarrassed. Amusingly, Judith had started to sing songs relating to speech that was being said. For example, one sunny day after a lovely afternoon with my parents in the garden, they were leaving to return home. Our driveway led out onto a small country lane, and Nigel, usually gave them the "all clear" to pull off the driveway and into the lane. On this particular instance, my father was revving the engine to pull out, when a motorcycle came into view. Immediately Nigel put the two palms of his hand up to my father and shouted "STOP'. Judy wound down the window and sang, 'Stop in the name of love, before you break my heart'. She got out of the car and then started singing and dancing to this song, in the lane. We all started to laugh and she was delighted by our reactions and was hysterical with laughter.

Perhaps one of the most noticeable and disturbing starts to Judy's behavioural changes was one day as she was driving the car, when my father, Nigel and myself were all present. The mountain road that we were travelling along, had many twists and turns. It is the Isle of Man's quickest road to travel along, with no enforcement of a speed limit. As we approached a tight bend at an all too fast speed, my father, Nigel and myself all shouted for Judy to slow down. At our alarming instructions, she hit the brakes at a very heavy rate, but managed to remain in control of the situation. We all looked at each other, eyes wide, but said nothing, yet a few yards further along Judith started to cry and then pulled the car over and asked Nigel to drive.

Secretly, my father had been trying to regain Judy's confidence in her driving ability, by giving her driving lessons in an unused, private car park. It was her sense of direction and getting lost that were causing her to lose faith in her driving skills. Anxiety and worry had set in. She had then just panicked at even the thought of driving the car. Judy had once been a very confident and outgoing person. Sometimes the life and soul of the party, and at other times very feisty and self-opinionated, but always full of her own ability to overcome adversity and problems. Yet everyday chores were becoming a difficulty for her. On one occasion, Judith and Jim had invited their two nephews, along with me and Nigel to lunch one day. The table was beautifully set with a white linen cloth and napkins with an array of condiments and breads to accompany the meal. We were all a little perplexed through the meal, as the food never seemed appropriate, or enough of it, but it wasn't until later when my cousins had left that myself and Nigel found food still in the oven and in the fridge, that should have been served at the lunch. When we raised the issue and commented to my mother, she was at first angry which quickly transcended into tears and anxiety. It was truly disturbing to witness. My father refused to entertain and invite any guests from that day onwards. It was clear that Judy was struggling with organizational skills at this point.

My parents' bungalow was on a small estate, very rural, but not far from the village centre. All the houses were bungalows and a high population of retired people lived there, although there were an increasing number of young families arriving. Their house had once been immaculate. The garden had been almost paradise. Totally private at the rear of the property. My father once had an aviary full of budgerigar with both an indoor and an outdoor area for them. In the centre of the garden was a beautiful pond with a Japanese-style bridge over and an ornamental waterfall. Trellising and a paved seating area separated the garden from the orchard. The orchard was planted with apple trees, pear trees, blackcurrant bushes, redcurrant bushes, strawberry plants, gooseberry bushes, potatoes, onions, garlic and peas. This trellising around the seating areas was smothered with climbing plants, with such an array of colour and smells in the mid-summer. The pond was full of koi carp. A joy to feed them from the ornamental bridge. Their little faces all appearing as soon as a footstep was on the bridge. Their tiny hungry mouths opening and closing in hurried anticipation. Two regal Manx palm trees stood at the property side of the garden adding a warm exotic appearance to the plot. The budgerigars added to the ambience with their busy, loud chatter and whistling.

Now, as we arrived outside my parents' house, upon walking past their immaculate trimmed front hedge, an excited barking could be heard from their little dog, Kana – an adorable brindle and cream long-haired, fan-tailed Chihuahua, who was in truth a little too stout and large to be a fully-fledged pedigree Chihuahua, yet full of cheekiness, cuteness and personality, reserved for that breed of dog. She was a full-time companion for my mother, Judith, who insisted the dog went everywhere with her – often tucked under her arm. This caused many an argument with shop workers who insisted that no dogs were allowed in the shop, even if it was being carried and "off the floor".

I knocked twice on the white uPVC front door, (the dog went into a frenzy), and I walked straight into the lounge, greeted by a frenetic grinning Chihuahua. I immediately noticed that my father looked grey in the face and immensely tired. While he was seated in his chair I went over and looked him in the eyes and asked him how he felt. His speech was slow and slurred; one of his pupils in his eye appeared to be dilated and very glassy-looking. My mother was not overly concerned and even appeared cheery. She already had her coat on and asked if we were going now. Despite my mother's reluctance, we persuaded her to leave the dog at home and the dog was more than happy with that arrangement when rewarded with a biscuit or two.

It was at this point when my father struggled to get out of his chair, and started to walk, that it was evident from the dragging and curling of his left foot, that he had most probably had a stroke. My husband, Nigel, drove us all to the doctor's surgery – a five minute journey that seemed to take forever. When we arrived, we helped my father out of the car, then we all waited in the reception area. I quietly explained to the receptionist that we suspected that my father had suffered a stroke. It was not his normal G.P., but they called my father in immediately. Nigel and I waited in the reception. My mother clumsily aided and chaperoned my father into the doctor's room.

The waiting room was drab, with lots of notices warning of all types of illnesses – heart attacks; strokes; diabetes; cirrhosis – the list was endless. The fluorescent tube lighting was harsh, and the receptionists were all babbling away on the telephone, or with patients. A small child was scraping a chair across the floor by pushing it.

My heart was racing; my head was pounding and my mouth was uncomfortably dry.

A few moments later, the doctor came bursting out of his room, heading straight for us, with a severe expression on his face. He explained abruptly and borderline accusingly, that my father had definitely suffered a stroke; that an ambulance had been called and that he had just given my father half an aspirin. He informed us in no uncertain terms that my father should have been taken by ambulance this morning. Any damage was likely to be irreversible by now. My mother was unusually calm and we asked her to travel in our car and explained that we would then go to the hospital later, after Jim had been formally admitted and settled in at the ward.

2
The Awakening

It was starting to sink in now. My mother would have to stay with us again. She more often than not, wandered at nighttime. Previously, she had frequently ended up in a neighbour's house after midnight with her coat on wanting to go shopping and rambling to herself, or an imaginary person. The neighbours were aware of Judith's condition and would bring her back to my father and settle her in. My parents were very fortunate to have such good neighbours. These wanderings were despite Judith taking Chloral Betaine 707mg for some time now, but she still awoke most nights, talking and confused. This proved startling and distressing for my father. On occasions during these times, she had insisted that my father take her shopping. In desperation my father would show her that it was dark outside, yet she would say that he was being ridiculous and that he was attempting to keep her captive in her own home.

The last time that my mother had stayed with us was some six months earlier, back in March 2011, after my father had suffered a seizure, which would later prove to have been a stroke, or series of strokes. Back then, myself and my husband had just returned from our annual holiday to South Goa, India. It was a place that we adored due to its beautiful scenery; the tranquility; the stunning, relatively quiet beaches and of course, the culture in India. We normally went there at the beginning of the New Year and returned mid-March, in time for plenty of hard work prior to opening the guest house to visitors. During this time in India we had managed to carry on taking bookings by email, and we would pick up the answer phone machine messages and return those calls. Thankfully and amazingly, we had never double booked any rooms.

On returning from our holiday in March 2011, we had then decided to celebrate by taking my parents out for a meal at our local eatery, called the "Creg-ny-Baa"; famous for its spectacular position on the T.T. Course (the famous motorcycle race on the Isle of Man), along with the fabulous views from the elevated and exposed position. My mother had been very excited at the prospect of going out to dine and she was receptive to the idea of leaving the dog at our house for the duration of the meal. Part of her dementia had led to her being overly outgoing and enthusiastically friendly, in a manner normally reserved for long-lost friends. This on occasions confused people with a definite, "Who are you?" quizzical look about them. People clearly questioned themselves, as to whether they knew Judith or not.

My mother had been most courteous to the staff at the restaurant back then and was full of laughs and smiles. With a little prompting and encouragement, she had managed to choose the famous fish and chips that the establishment served. We had sat at a bay window table, from where we looked out to sea, over agricultural land and green fields. I remember the two reservoirs nearby had shone like blue topaz in the dazzling sun, and the delicious smell of food had drifted into the corner, where we were sitting. Just enough to increase the appetite. My father had seemed a little quiet and slow, perhaps troubled or tired, I had thought. He had ordered a pint of lager with his meal, despite him relaying that he had not had a drink since Christmas. He later failed to finish his drink, and indeed his meal. He had apologised for not being hungry. My mother had a dessert – they were her favourite part of any meal. I recall her grinning with delight as she was eating it and had tried to tempt us all with a spoonful of her chocolate fudge cake. After devouring it, we had then decided that we would have a coffee back down at our house. We all had snippets of food wrapped in serviettes for the dog. This was the very least that Kana would expect upon our return. Very undignified, but necessary.

It was as we had sat in the lounge back at our house, having our coffee and chatting, that I had noticed my father acting strangely; his face suddenly went completely blank and his eyes appeared glazed, dilated and fixed into a stare. He had then slumped to his left hand side and started shaking slightly from his head down, while his left arm was curled under and clamped to his chest. Immediately I had rang for an ambulance which arrived soon after and took him to the hospital. This was the first instance back then, when my mother had needed to stay with us.

So here we were again, in very similar circumstances. My mother would need to stay with us in the meantime. She was currently on a waiting list to be formally assessed at a government-run unit for dementia, and other such illnesses, at the Elderly Mentally Infirm Unit. My mother's assigned care worker, was a small, blonde Scottish lady, called Marie. She had kept explaining to my father, who would ring up for help in dealing with my mother, that Judith was getting closer to the top of the list. He had asked for help numerous times with my mother's nocturnal escapades, as he was struggling to cope, or even sleep. Judith was constantly becoming upset and tearful too.

This time, after Jim was whisked off in the ambulance from the G.P.'s surgery, we drove back to our house in Onchan, but only after we had collected belongings from my parents' house for both Jim in hospital and for Judith's stay at our house. As we got out of the car on our driveway, my mother thanked us very much for a lovely day out, and then said that she was very worried about Jim, her husband. My mother was clearly unsure about the events that had just taken place. I had to explain to her that Jim had gone to the hospital, as the doctor believed that he had suffered a stroke, and that we would visit him in hospital later, yet it was still questionable as to whether she comprehended the gravity of the situation. Inside the house we made a cold drink and sat with it out in the garden, by the rockery, listening to the birds singing and chirping and watching the honeybees and bumble bees buzzing in and out of the lavender bushes. The house was enclosed by trees all around – Sycamore; Elm; Oak, Larchwood to name but a few. The different shades of green were breathtaking. One couldn't help but be soul-soothed by the setting. I was trying my best to keep my mother distracted from thinking about my father. She seemed relaxed and cheery though.

Later, I made a simple pizza and salad for tea. My mother ate all of it, with no hesitation and opted for an ice cream after. It was at this point that I fetched the light green box that we had recovered from my parents' house earlier. It contained her medication, all in pre-made separate sections, compiled by the pharmacy. They were divided into morning tablets/mid-morning/lunchtime/afternoon/evening/bedtime. The tablets were so numerous that I was taken aback and wondered how she could be monitored for side-effects, or alternatively, which tablets were benefiting her? I asked Nigel to see the medication too. My husband reassured me that the doctors dealt with this illness on a regular basis. I felt the tiny hairs on the back of my neck prickle and a wave of anxiety wash over me. Something disturbed me about these number of pills, but surely Nigel must be right. My immediate response, which was of anger, would not help matters. I needed to try and keep it together. Any outbursts from me might be detrimental to my mother's care, I felt. Judith was so adept at taking the pills and took one mouthful of water to wash them down. Judith sat in the kitchen, while Nigel and I cleared the dinner plates and filled the dishwasher. We then all went to sit in the television lounge. The news was on. My mother started laughing at the news. It was neither funny, or appropriate to laugh, but she carried on.; all of the while twisting tissues and plastic bags that she had stashed in her handbags. My father had explained previously that Judy would wrap things up in tissues, like her wedding ring and other jewellery. He therefore had to unwrap all tissues prior to disposing of them.

When we explained to my mother that we would go and visit Jim after she had used the bathroom, she was almost child-like in her excitement, and followed me quickly upstairs to use the bathroom. Before leaving for the hospital, Judith insisted on bringing all five handbags with her too, that she had reclaimed on our earlier visit to her house. She just would not relent on this, no matter how much coaxing we tried. She became more and more disturbed and anxious at the prospect of leaving the handbags behind. To calm matters down we just took them and loaded them into the car. For once Judith had forgotten that the dog was still lying on the couch, and no persuasion on our part was needed to leave Kana behind.

On the way to the hospital Judith started to tell us how horrid Jim was to her and how he wanted to hurt her. She kept telling us what a nasty man he was. I was very confused by this. Was it the dementia, or was she confiding in us? To this day, I have no answers to this. Was she imagining this, or was my father becoming irritated by her increasingly difficult disposition? I will never know.

Arriving at the hospital Judith became very cheerful again and greeted everybody that passed her by, as if they were old acquaintances. It was a little embarrassing, but very comical to watch peoples' expressions.

The hospital was modern with an impressive glass frontage and large revolving doors that you had to step between whilst they moved forward. They were both time consuming and unnecessary, but great fun. Judith was galloping into them like a horse. We humoured her by making quiet naying noises, being careful not to catch anybody's attention. This proved to be a bad move. All the way up to the ward where my father was, my mother was galloping and naying, while crying hysterically with laughter. We were like the parents of a hyperactive toddler, also loaded-up with two of her handbags each.

On reaching the ward, my mother had personally greeted everybody in the male unit, which consisted of perhaps six beds in total, before she went and hugged my father. It was at this point that Judith became concerned for him and a little tearful. She sat down beside him and held his hand. She would take huge sighs and say, "Oh Jim". I went to speak with the Sister in charge of the ward. She confirmed my fears, that my father had suffered a stroke. More tests and scans were to be performed the following day. (These went on to show that he had suffered previous smaller strokes).

We visited my father at least once a day, but normally twice per day in the following days. Having my mother staying with us highlighted the immense difficulties that my father must have been experiencing whilst trying to cope with my mother's care.

This day, I had managed to calm my mother when she first awoke very early. I persuaded her to part with her coat and shoes, undress and go back to sleep, until a more reasonable hour of the morning. Later, after waking again I made her the usual porridge and a cup of tea, which she had while sitting up in bed, with the television on. Following that, the green plastic box with the plethora of medication was brought out, and after some persuasion Judith took them – impressively all in one go. One handful of tablets – one sip of water again and they were all gone.

Later that morning I was to take my mother to the Day Care Centre not far from my parents' house, but before this I placed a clean flannel, a fresh bar of soap and a fluffy white towel on the bed and asked Judith if she would take a shower before going, and brush her teeth.

Fifteen minutes later I popped back in to check on my mother. Judith had brushed her teeth, but her mood had changed drastically. Her face was visibly angry. I asked her if something was wrong. It was like lighting a fuse. The torrent of abuse was unprecedented and appeared out of nowhere. My mother's language had never been foul before the dementia, even when she had lost her temper. Yet now, every other word was swearing and cursing. I calmly attempted to ask her if she wanted a shower, but this led to accusations of calling her dirty and filthy. I suggested going back to her house in Ramsey to get freshened up in the bathroom there. I thought maybe familiarity would help in this situation. She calmed immediately and agreed that she would like that. She instantly apologised but told me that I was still "a bit of a fucking witch", and chuckled.

Half an hour later we were travelling in the car over the mountain singing, "She'll be Coming Around the Mountain When She Comes". My parent's house and our house lay approximately twelve miles apart. The quickest route from ours was to take the very scenic mountain road – the most exciting part of the famous T.T. motorcycle race. Sadly, also a circuit that had claimed many lives, both young and not so young. Bunches of flowers and small crosses or memorials were evident whilst travelling along this route, signifying the very fine line between those that succeeded in completing the course and those that fatally failed, in any given split second. The mountain road can be breathtakingly beautiful on a clear sunny day. Hills, green valleys and fields bordered by the contrasting blue sea. White fluffy sheep appeared as big as clouds, dotting the green fields. The odd bird of prey hovering above, with crows and seagulls riding the thermals. Most notable on the mountain road, is the "no speed limit", – at all. The travelling time could take anywhere between twenty minutes to forty five minutes, dependent on the amount and type of traffic in front. The biggest hindrance was often the near juggernaut of a vehicle; the Co-Op lorry. Too long to overtake safely and too wide for many parts of the road also.

On parking outside of my mother's house, she thanked me profusely and told me what a super day out she had and insisted that we must do it again soon. She gave me a big hug and a kiss. I thanked her too but explained that I was coming in with her to her house. She thanked me further.

The house was now grim from outside. The once beauty of it had long gone and was left to neglect and darkness. The front garden was becoming overgrown. The compulsive collection of garden fairies were now lying broken – limbless, headless or wingless. The brightly coloured painted plant pots had faded and paint was peeling off them. An irrational collection of beach boulders had been randomly placed around the entrance porch, next to the fairies. The blinds and curtains were constantly closed, be it day or night. Inside the house was gloomy and cluttered. The air smelled musty, mouldy and dank. The coffee table, which had once lain bare was covered with items wrapped in tissues or wrapped in plastic bags. Coasters were spread out in an orderly manner, each with a random item placed on display.

Items included rings, paperclips, coins, scissors, small ornaments or cutlery. Plastic bags were stuffed in every crevice of the sofa. Again, these would contain items wrapped up in tissues. Newspapers overflowed everywhere. Judy would not allow Jim to throw anything out. He had to "secretly", go to the dustbin to discard rubbish, otherwise my mother would start going through the dustbin, convinced that he was discarding her valuables. Everywhere was dirty and dusty. A once immaculate house had layers of dust covering the ornaments and furniture. The house now smelled stale and old. Perhaps the house was kept so dark for that reason. Unable to be seen by my parents themselves or by the outside world. Even the dog was scratching constantly. My parents appeared to be virtual prisoners in their own home.

I had been too busy with the guesthouse to notice what was really happening with my parents. When I saw them during the season, it was generally when they visited us, and, when the weather was fine, we would all sit in the garden. Judith loved the glen and the garden. The dog would become giddy and zoom around the garden with a manic grin on her dear little face. My father had successfully managed to keep the full extent of my mother's dementia hidden. We knew that certain aspects of her personality had changed. She had always been very house-proud and the garden was immaculate. My mother was always well groomed – her make-up was always perfect and her hair always curled. Sadly, these were attributes of the past now.

Inside the house I asked my mother if she was able to get washed herself. She said that she could but wanted her hair washing. She asked me if I could do this for her. I replied that I would wash her hair after she'd had a wash. As I watched her expression it became obvious to me that she could not recall which of the rooms was the bathroom. To reassure her, I said that we would both go into the bathroom and check that there was some soap and fresh towels. I then left her to get washed and to brush her teeth again. I walked out of the bathroom and back into the lounge. My eyes welled up – the sadness of the situation hit me at full pelt. The enormity of the disease had only just started. When Judith eventually came out of the bathroom she looked relieved to see me and rushed over to thank me for coming over. She then commenced to inform me that something terrible had happened to Jim, and that Jim was dead. I hastened to explain that Jim was not dead but was in hospital after having a stroke. She nonchalantly said that was good and asked if we could visit him to bring him some sweets. I explained that I would wash her hair for her, but evidently that moment had gone, and there was no persuading her to go back in the bathroom to do so. I told her that we would go and visit Jim a little later on, but firstly we would go to the Day Care Centre and see Bridget, her friend, who was in fact the Senior Care Assistant at the unit. The Day Care Centre was only a five minute drive away from my parents' house by car. We went through the estate, passed by their doctors' surgery and passed by the cottage hospital, then a little further up the hill. From here you could see the beautiful man-made lake of Mooragh Park, with all of its glorious garden reflected in the glass-like water. A small road separated the park from the sea front and the beauty of the Irish Sea. The view was magnificent and many Victorian houses had been built taking full advantage of this view. We parked outside the Unit and my mother grabbed my hand and held on to it while we went through the Day Care Centre door. Judith was breaking into a near run. The lady in charge, Bridget appeared. There was a brief exchange of introductions and my mother insisted that I was her sister. – neither Bridget nor I corrected her. Judith then went off holding Bridget's hand and waving goodbye with a wide cheery smile. It was a weirdly reminiscent scenario of dropping my daughter off at playschool, decades ago. I then headed back to the car and drove back over the mountain, for a few hours back at my house.

Due to my mother's severe mood changes in the morning when she was left alone (not long after her medication), my husband and myself had taken it in turns to sit with Judith and get showered and ready ourselves, at different times. It was exhausting both physically and emotionally, but this saved Judith flying into a foul mood, accusing us of all sorts of plotting and sabotage. It stopped these mood swings and the consequent running around the house rattling windows, banging on doors and windows, and shouting for Jim. She was like a person possessed and these moods came on so quickly. They seemed to graduate roughly half an hour to an hour after taking her medication in the morning, and as fast as half an hour after the meds at night. Nighttime were the worst episodes. My mother was seeing things, people and animals. Her bedroom at our house had two large windows. One large window facing the front aspect of the house overlooking the formal garden and rockery, then down to the stream. The second smaller window was an arched long window overlooking the cobbled parking area and into the trees. The high double bed was in the middle of the room against the back wall. There was a separate en-suite toilet and shower room. Each night Judith would insist that some people were gathered outside wanting to break in, or she would fret that the "children" were left outside in the garden to the front and would be angry at our cruelty of leaving them outside. I attempted to reassure her by telling her that nobody was there. This was not the best tactic, I soon learnt. She would accuse me of lying and trying to keep her prisoner. She told me that the people were going to break in, and that I was so stupid that I couldn't see that. I tried my hardest, but I couldn't and didn't know how to deal with the outbursts.

I was trying my hardest to stay positive, but between having my mother staying, which was a full-time job in itself, then worrying and visiting my father in hospital, it was very difficult to stay focused on remaining positive. Sleeping at night was now a problem, not just for my mother, but for me now, too. I felt that I was just nervous sleeping, waking up through the night feeling anxious and panicked, waiting for my mother to bang on the door, or to wake up to her shouting. She actually frightened me. She was unpredictable and unrecognisable at times. The word "demented" had never been more aptly used. It felt like a rollercoaster ride that I wanted to stop.

When the time came to pick up my mother from the Day Care Centre, I got into the car and put the radio on. It was another beautiful day with clear blue skies. A good sing-along in the car on the way over left me feeling happier and more relaxed by the time I arrived at Ramsey. The Senior Care Worker, Bridget, at the Day Care Centre, explained that Judith was rather up and down in her mood, but more disturbingly, Judith had told her that my father, Jim, had died. Bridget had explained to my mother that he was only in hospital, but Judith was adamant that he had died. When my mother saw me she was tearful, until I told her that we would go straight over and visit Jim, who was not dead, but in hospital and poorly. All the way back over the mountain, she repeated how much she loved Jim.

After a very quick dash back to my house to pick up some necessary clean pyjamas and underwear for my father, we then travelled to the hospital. Judith was getting very anxious on the way and kept telling me that the "children" had been left alone at the house. I explained that the dog (which I thought may have been "the children"), was at home with Nigel. She started shouting, saying that he (Nigel), had better not take the dog out in the rain, (a battle we regularly had). The dog would often be desperate to go out, yet my mother ordered and threatened us not to take her out in the rain. We usually managed distraction techniques and took Kana for a stroll up the lane. I then had to try and sneak back into the house and try to towel-dry the dog if it was raining, before it leapt back onto the couch with Judith. Naturally, my mother would notice that the dog was damp, and call me all the names under the sun for around five or ten minutes.

Both myself and Nigel agreed that my mother needed some professional evaluation as to what was going on with her dementia, which would be the only way to also see what was happening with her medication. We hoped, as my father had, that my mother was somewhere near the top of the "waiting list", for that. Anytime not spent with my mother, for instance, when she was left watching the television while we prepared food, meant her mood would change. She would accuse us of planning something; of keeping her captive and removing her from "the children". I had started waking up during the night, sobbing uncontrollably – so uptight and nervous. My throat and chest tightened in a way that I had never experienced before. I needed to go to the G.P. myself. I was bleeding nearly continually for the whole month now and it had been getting much worse of late. Investigations were done some three years ago, but all the tests proved clear, with nothing abnormal being found. I hoped that this bleeding would settle down soon. Every week I expected it to cease, but it never seemed to.

Upon our arrival into the hospital car park my mother had calmed down at the prospect of taking Jim some sweets. We both went into the little shop in the foyer of the hospital. My mother's eyes lit up and she raced towards the sweets and continued to inspect all of the confectionary. We ended up taking five packets of sweets, as Judith could not decide which ones he would prefer. Judith ran to Jim in a very dramatic manner, as we entered the ward with him lying in bed. My father beamed back at her, trying to say, "Oh my Judy", as he normally did. Yet, when she reached his bed, she near ignored him and picked up his drink of squash and drank it down in one, slamming the cup down on the over-bed table, like a spaghetti-western whisky-drinking baddie. She began laughing and enjoying the attention. It transpired after talking to a nurse, that my father would be in hospital for some time, but he would move to the rehabilitation ward, where most severe stroke patients would end up at some point. As he presented at the time, he could not feed himself or hold a cup. He had been left so weak by the stroke. He could barely walk either, yet he seemed reasonably aware of his situation and seemed even rather relieved to get some sleep. I truly believed that his strokes were brought about by the sheer exhaustion of looking after my mother with dementia. Her moods were all over the place. Lucid one moment, then totally confused and angry the next, tinged with suspicion and accusations.

I felt so immensely sorry for both of them yet was I helpless to improve their situations myself.

3

The Cloud Form

The changing moment followed a particularly bad Saturday night, after my mother had taken her medication. I had settled her down in bed, put the light on in the en-suite for her and partially closed that door, in the hope that if she awoke during the night, then the guiding light should help her to the bathroom. We kissed goodnight and I pulled her bedroom door to.

Nigel had poured me a glass of red wine and we sat discussing the day's events. Maybe half an hour had passed, when we heard my mother coming down the stairs. She burst into the lounge and said how dare I lock her in the bedroom. I was a "spiteful fucking bitch", and she wasn't going to stand for it any longer. I explained that the door wasn't locked, but was only pulled to, to stop Shani the cat from jumping on her bed. She replied that she was going out for the night, stormed out to the front door, which was locked for the night, and after trying the door, began kicking it and screaming. I kept out of the way, as I was clearly her main focus of upset. Nigel tried to calm her down and offered her a coffee. She started to accuse him of lying and being on "their side", and that he had stopped her from seeing "the children". We gently persuaded her to sit down in the lounge, with a packet of crisps and a glass of water, until she started to get sleepy. At which point I managed to get her to hold my hand, and we climbed the stairs together.

I hardly slept that night. My nerves were shattered. Every time I woke up during the night, I woke up crying. I was a complete mess and was beyond coping.

The next morning, I got up filled with the dread of having a day like the previous. I made the porridge for my mother as normal, along with a cup of tea, all followed by the array of tablets. It was a wet day and rather windy. The trees in the glen were swaying and sometimes creaking, the house was tucked into a narrow valley and was totally sheltered from the winds normally. The rain nearly always came straight down unless a storm had whipped up. When the rain eased a little, I crept out to take the dog out. As I did so, we had evidently been spotted, as my mother hammered on the window furiously and screamed at me to get the dog in, out of the rain. My mother's face at the window was wild and seething. Her green eyes flashing with anger. I hoped that by the time the dog and I returned, she would have forgotten and simmered down somewhat. We trotted up the lane in the spitting rain. The trees were naturally all bent in towards the road on either side and provided a near-covered walkway. The birds were still singing despite the drizzle. Little Kana did the necessaries and we ran back down to the house. The stream at the bottom of the garden was now a river and roared away, muddy and brown. My heart was racing at the thought of facing my mother. We walked past the lounge window and I peered through the white butterfly-pattern net curtains. I could see my mother seated on the couch watching the television. I crept in through the door quietly. I picked up the dog and carried her upstairs to where the "wet dog" towel was. She was immediately giddy and started darting from side to side barking. She then turned and galloped downstairs. I tried to grab her tail, but I missed. My heart sank. The next thing I heard was, "Jesus Christ this dog is bloody soaking. You evil, evil, little bitch. This dog does not go out when it's raining .... ". The air was blue and the torrent of verbal abuse unrelenting. I went into the living room and explained that the dog was desperate to go out to the toilet. I had clearly raised my voice, unintentionally, but I had. She told me to stop shouting at her; told me I was a "bossy fucking bitch", and tried to throw her water at me. She told me to leave ***her*** house and said that I had always caused trouble between her and her mother. I was to leave ***her*** house now. I was once again a "scheming fucking witch". As I went to leave the lounge she lunged at me and gripped me by the throat with both hands. She looked me straight in the eyes and was biting her lips as her hands pressed harder. Nigel knocked into us as he opened the lounge door. I ran straight out into the garden and burst into a cry. I couldn't cope with this. I didn't have the knowledge or experience to be able to handle my mother. She had always been a feisty lady and a tad argumentative, but this was a different kettle of fish altogether.

My mother was banging on the kitchen window shouting again. Where she had once calmed down when Nigel intervened, this was no longer happening. I honestly felt that I was on the parapet of a breakdown. I needed to run away, or just slip away. My own mental health was fragile – I could not cope.

For a moment I stood still, gazing at all of the beauty that filled the garden and thought of all the wonderful things that life had to offer. The flowers and the bees; the stunning green trees and the birds; my pretty little cat and the gorgeous little dog; the river and the baby trout that we often saw; the tranquil scenic walks in the glen and the beaches they often led to. I wiped my eyes and blew my nose. I collected my thoughts and realised at that precise moment, that I could not cope. Period.

I calmly walked back into the house. By now my mother was watching television again, with the damp dog across her lap. She was now laughing again, in a childish carefree manner. I spoke with my husband, and told him that I had made a decision to ring the assessment unit at the Mental Health Services and ask them to take my mother immediately, as I could not deal with the situation as it was. My mother needed professional help. Nigel sat with Judith while I rang them to explain that my mother needed help and equally important, was the fact that I could not manage her and was not willing to cope any longer. Professional help was desperately needed. They explained to me that they couldn't just admit her – it wasn't that easy. If my mother refused to go with them voluntarily, then the next step was a mental health section 2 and that would take hours to implement.; there were just not the two doctors on duty needed to do this. In addition, there were no beds available. I stood my ground. My father had suffered two strokes while awaiting their help. I too could not cope. I was crying yet again while pleading with them. I reverted to threatening to drive my mother to the hospital and leaving her there. Dirty tactics but needs must. They would ring me back in five minutes.

Sure enough, five minutes later they rang me, and told me that there would be a free bed now. They had moved another resident who was due for release. They would come and collect Judith, and they hoped that she would go with them off her own accord. In the meantime, I was to collect her things together.

Guilt flowed over me – I kept thinking that what I was doing was heartless – I had failed my mother. Yet the situation that we were in was not sustainable and Judith really did require specialist help, to make any progress with having her moods stabilised, along with alleviating the hallucinations with "the children". I was at my wits end. My nerves were shattered. My mother and I had always had a difficult and sometimes turbulent relationship, as far back as I could remember. This in itself made the scenario we were in very difficult. We had never had a hands-on physical bond. Any physical contact had been kept to a minimum, adding to my alien understanding of my mother's needs. I proceeded to pack Judith's toiletries into a green and navy canvas overnight bag – soap, flannels, towels, underwear, nightgown, deodorant, socks and clean clothes. As I was packing them my mother came into the room. She calmly asked me, "Are they coming to take me? Have you rang those people?". I explained that these people were going to help her. It would be like going to a hotel for a little while, as Jim was in hospital and the doctor needed to look at her medication and maybe change it. While she was in there I would look after Kana and bring her in to visit.

The explosion was instant. "I am not fucking mad you know. You think I am mental, but I'm not. You're the one who is fucking mental not me". The torrent of abuse and foul language was unheard of from my mother pre-dementia. She was screaming and threatening, but in an almost overly dramatic manner. Almost like a toddler seeking attention and behaving badly to an audience. The screaming continued and she began kicking doors and banging on windows. Shani the cat shot up the stairs towards the bedroom, looking petrified. I followed her up and stooped to collect her in my arms to reassure her. Kana hurried up the stairs with her tail between her legs, looking perturbed. I closed the bedroom door behind us and made sure it was safely locked. I sat crying on the bed with the cat and the dog. Tears quietly streaming down my face. I could hear my mother banging on the windows and doors, screaming and shouting profanities. My head felt like it was going to burst from the pressure of it all.

Nigel was at this point out in the garage, which was situated in outbuildings away from the house. I was willing him back in. Any doubts I had about questioning the need for the assessment unit dissolved completely. I waited for silence for ten minutes and then crept downstairs. My mother was sitting on the sofa twisting tissues and stuffing them into the handbags. I said hello and asked her if she would like a drink of water. She replied, "That would be nice". I got a cold glass of water from the fridge and placed it on the table for her, then we sat in the lounge together, watching television. The moods swings were like a light switch – on and off, that quickly.

Sometime later, a car drove on to the parking area. Out of the car stepped my mother's assigned Care Worker, Marie, with another lady with long medium brown hair, tied back in a ponytail. She wore a severe, harsh expression and had thin angry lips. I went to the door and let them in. I firstly apologised for the trouble that I was causing them, but explained, through tears, that I felt that my mother really needed some professional help, as I couldn't cope with her outbursts and mood swings. I explained the sudden changes that appeared after taking some of her medication.

Their faces looked daggers at me. Their expressions clearly thought that I was either lying, or exaggerating. Only time would tell.

I handed Marie the overnight bag and my mother's handbags too. She accepted them and glowered at me. No hint of a smile. My mother went off, hand in hand with Marie, like a kid being taken to a foster home. They drove off along the green, leafy, arched-tree lane. I felt numb and surreal-like; almost like a nightmare that I was waiting to wake up from. I climbed the stairs in a state of shock – I felt sick. I lay down on the bed and broke into an uncontrollable sob, like a distressed baby, then cried myself to sleep.

I woke up with a fright, as Nigel was shaking my shoulder. I had no idea at this point if it was morning or night, but it was dark. He explained that I would have to get up if I wanted to visit my father in hospital. My heart sank as the dawn of reality hit me again. My mind raced around haphazardly; how was my mother? Was she settled in? Was she frightened and worried? How could I have done that to my mother? Now I would have to tell my father. Would he be angry or very upset? Most of all, would he understand why I had to do this? I jumped off the bed with a wave of anxiety filling my heavy, pounding head. I must take the little dog for a walk; she will be desperate to go out.

Nigel opened the bedroom door wider, holding a wide-grinning Chihuahua. Her legs were doggy-paddling in mid-air to get to me. Nigel placed her on the bed, and she began to zoom around it playfully, stopping every few seconds with her paws down, and her tail and bottom in the air, clearly filled with mischief. I noticed at this point that she was a damp dog – she had been out for a walk – Nigel had taken her. I was thankful for that. I played with Kana for a little while, freshened up and then Nigel and myself headed out to the car.

It was a dark night and very windy. Leaves were shed over the road; branches littered the gullies and pavements. When we got to the ward that my father was on, we found that he was not where he should have been; the bed he had occupied was empty. My heart missed a beat and jumped up to my throat. One of the nurses must have seen my face, as she came rushing over. She informed me that my father had now been moved to the rehabilitation ward. She explained that all the necessary tests had been completed and that there was nothing else medically that they could do for him on this current ward.

The rehab unit, better known as the dreaded, "Ward 20", was just a five-minute drive away. It was a matter of perhaps 500 metres away only, from the unit where my mother was being assessed. We parked immediately outside of Ward 20 in the allocated tarmac parking area, neatly divided into staff and visitors parking lots. There were grass lawns surrounding the building, and wild rabbits were lazily gnawing away at it, totally un-phased by the comings and goings of the ward traffic. A few rooks were digging deep for worms submerging their huge beaks into the freshly mown turf.

As we approached the entrance, we came upon a middle-aged man with only one leg, sitting in a wheelchair, smoking a cigarette. He looked unkempt with peppery grey hair, shoulder length which was pulled back into a ponytail. We smiled and acknowledged him. He smiled back with a wide beaming grin, exposing his rotten and missing teeth. He looked like a Fagan-type character; mischievous, with some good tales to tell. The glass doors automatically parted as we approached them, revealing a vending machine, packed with crisps, sweets, chocolate bars and cans of drinks. Maybe it was the crock of gold goal that was being aimed for when undergoing vigorous rehabilitation. The ultimate unhealthy reward – a trip to the vending machine.

We carried on along the corridor until we reached the "nurses' station". It was manned by a plump, homely-looking nurse and one rather skinny, effeminate male nurse. We enquired about my father. They jokingly referred to him as the "new inmate".

The bay that my father was in had four beds on each side. All were male patients and all probably seventy years of age or more – some missing limbs and all pretty much bed bound. My father was pleased to see us and asked us how he had ended up in "this dump". He couldn't recall having a stroke and was unaware of his predicament. I nervously waited to try and explain to him that I had requested my mother to be placed at the assessment unit (for which she was waiting), for professional help. Eventually, when I explained it to him, my father seemed rather surprised. He explained that he had indeed being trying for ages to get that assessment for her, but to no avail. He was happy enough with the decision and agreed that it would be beneficial for her, although he still seemed insensitive and curt in his manner, probably due to the mixture of him suffering from the stroke and the recent medication being prescribed.

The relief of hearing this from my father was immense. I tried my hardest not to shed a tear – tears of both sadness and relief again – but it was not to be. I shirked them off, attempted a brave smile for my father, and headed off to the vending machine for a tearful moment to myself.

Of all the vending machines that I have ever encountered, I have never before found one that contained Jelly Tots. My absolute favourites. I put my coins into the slot and watched the small yellow packet of a sure sugar hit, slide forward and politely drop the delicate packet of joy into the stainless-steel container. I pushed the plastic lid in and scooped up my prize. I stood back and studied the contents of the machine once more. There on the top shelf were two rows containing cans of coke. It was a long drop from the top shelf to the dispensing tray. I smiled to myself. Surely any person purchasing an item from the said machine wished to eat or drink the item almost immediately. I pictured buying a can for my father and pulling the ring to open it for him. This would be followed by a minor explosion and a significant shower of coke, engulfing all those present. Seriously, what kind of idiot..........?". I smiled to myself – there had been very little humour in the past week or so. I guessed the person filling the machine was having a bit of an inward joke, in an otherwise monotonous job.

I returned to the ward, (without the coke), and talked with my father, who was talking, secretly, about the other patients, in a slow, but rather too loud and inappropriate manner. "See him over there, he's a miserable old bugger, and his wife, well, she's a bit of a dolly bird, quite a lot younger than him I would say. Probably flattened a bit of ground in her time". OK, right, time to change the subject, and we started to drown poor father out, by talking over him. We switched the focus of the conversation back to how he was feeling. He explained that he was feeling fine and that he had no idea why he was in this awful place. He then started to tell me that my mother had been into visit him. Was this true, or was he becoming delirious?

I spoke with the Sister on the ward, who confirmed that this was in fact true. A Health Care Assistant had brought Judith over to see him. She explained to me that my mother had been very pleased to see him and had started crying when she had to leave him. So heart-breaking – forty eight years of marriage and then circumstances separate them. It must have been so difficult for them both. My father's stroke had changed his personality. He continued to emphasise that he didn't really understand why they bothered to bring Judy over – all she did was cry and she didn't bring anything with her. He relayed that the nurse had told him that stress can bring on strokes, and he explained that Judy crying for half an hour, while he was lying in bed was very stressful. My father must have known that Judith was in the Assessment Unit already, or maybe he was just not able to make sense of the situation, due to his stroke.

Nearly everyday somebody from the unit walked Judy over to see Jim from then on. On occasions, when I was already visiting, I would witness my mother arriving with a care worker. She was always holding their hand like a toddler, and her walk was more stooped and slower than it had ever been. My father with his new-found insensitivity following the stroke, would remark loudly, "Here comes Clyde" – a referral to the orangutan from the Clint Eastwood movie Every Which Way.

4

The Stream of Sunlight

After a few days of Judith settling into the assessment unit, myself and Nigel started to visit, (we had been in touch with the unit, who had advised us not to visit for a while).

I had been to the Mental Health Unit some years previously – not to the elderly side of it, but to the normal adult side. That had been some ten years ago, but nothing appeared to have changed. The nursing staff mainly sat in the glass office and the patients wandered around aimlessly and vacantly. To reach Judith's unit, we had to go through this adult part of the unit. There was a security entrance to go through, to access the first unit, with a signing-in book by the door to this. Staff in the glass office would then release the door from the confines of the glass office. Upon gaining access you would find yourself actually inside the patient area. We needed to walk through the dining area of this unit, then around a corner and along a corridor. The smell wafted around of cooked food, reminiscent of school dinner days. The paint was drab and the environment sterile and hospital-like. We reached another security door, but without the captive audience. To gain access you had to rely on catching a member of staff's eye, through the small square security glass panel, to request entry. Often my mother would be pacing up and down the corridor. If she spotted us, she would run excitedly to the door and begin pulling and yanking it frantically.

Each time we visited she would ask about Jim and become tearful. It was such a painful process, but one which we hoped would end in a few weeks following the professional assessment.

Some days we would venture out into the garden at the unit with my mother. The garden was partly paved and had lots of shrubbery, that provided camouflage for the birds. They pecked and flitted around the garden in blissful ignorance of the nature of their environment. Judy's face would light up when she spotted the birds. She had always loved animals and nature. She connected with it and had always appreciated nature's beauty. For her, nature seemed to soothe her soul. She was calm and at peace when alone with her natural environment. She never overlooked the beauty of a landscape, the serenity of the sea or the wonder of an animal. We would lead my mother around the garden, moving slowly so she could touch the plants and flowers. She would comment on how beautiful they were. The high metal fence around the garden was the only telling sign as to the type of establishment the garden belonged to.

Back inside the unit, the residents continued their relentless wandering, staring blankly into midair, rocking and talking to themselves. Perhaps, two healthcare assistants would sit accompanying the patients in the main lounge. Tea, coffee and biscuits would be offered regularly to both the patients and their visitors. There were two other quiet rooms in the unit; one with magazines, books and a bubble machine with changing colours, that was mesmerizing and relaxing. The other room with just seating and a table. Both rooms were strictly orderly with books stacked away in order of height and with magazines all placed in the rack. The corridor in the unit was long with a dado rail running along it. An occasional picture was safely screwed to the perfectly painted walls. On either side of the corridor were rooms. The first three rooms were the lounges. One of these was the main lounge with chocolate brown leather sofas and easy chairs, surrounded by a few coffee tables and the large television. The other two rooms were the quiet rooms. The next was an office with computers and desks for staff. A large bulky lady was usually there, with a severe short dyed-red haircut and a dark, intimidating expression – a member of staff, but who could have easily passed for a patient. Further along were the bedrooms at either side of the corridor, along with some toilets – all normally locked during the daytime. On the few times that I had asked my mother if she needed the toilet, I had to actively find a member of staff to either unlock the toilet or unlock Judy's en-suite room. I wondered how a confused dementia patient could find the bathroom, in a strange, new environment, when desperate. There were no signs or indications of a bathroom. Even the toilet door held no clue.

Every time I left the unit, I felt a sense of uneasiness, guilt and anxiety. There was an underlying fear of the unit merely coping with Judith, rather than helping or treating her, in any way. I never witnessed any patients engaged in activities, or any signs of their active engagement with members of staff. Yet there was no alternative place to seek treatment on such a small island. Either, we as a family coped with my mother, which ultimately, had already led to my father's stroke, or she came to the unit for professional assessment. No other private help would be appropriate, until the assessment was completed. The Mental Health Services had been involved with my parents, regarding my mother's dementia for getting on one year now. They managed to place my mother for a few hours at a day centre, for one day a week, and at a later date, two days per week, but my father had explained that he found coaxing Judy to get washed, dressed and ready so early in the morning more stressful than not going at all. She was a very strong-willed lady and would put up a good fight when confronted with doing something against her will. A consequence of all this stress had inevitably resulted in his suffering of a least one confirmed stroke, although later tests revealed multiple smaller earlier strokes. I was adamant that no further casualties should be inflicted – not on my health; not on my husband's health and not on our relationship.

My father was eventually released from the Rehabilitation Ward, but not before a personal alarm, worn around his neck was allocated, along with a direct dial telephone, and an alarm system that summoned assistance. My father's walking improved, and he appeared capable of driving again, (although we had reservations about this).

The support worker referred my father to the, "meals on wheels" people, who would deliver him one meal per day for a small cost. He was more than happy with the arrangements in place. We had a meeting with the care worker and the Mental Health Services, and we were all in agreement that my father could not provide full-time care for Judith any longer, as he was struggling to look after himself. Therefore, we came to the joint conclusion that my mother's best option was to move into a Residential Care Home facility. My father and myself agreed to jointly investigate the availability of such places. It felt so sad to be going down this route. I had failed my mother and my father was so frustrated by not being able to help her too. My father who was now seventy one years old appeared to be struggling with his own emotions and mental health too. My father would eventually, when recovered enough from his stroke, drive to see my mother at the assessment unit every day. I would try and meet up with him and visit on a daily basis too. Seeing my mother under such circumstances affected both myself and my father, but he was particularly affected. He was bitter and angry at the hand that life had now dealt him. He was almost in denial about how poorly Judith was and often accused her of, "putting it on". It was so sad to watch. My father and myself visited various care homes, looking for appropriate care that my mother might like, and that would be beneficial to her condition. Sadly, a couple of the most suitable care homes that appeared to have the best dementia facilities and trained staff, were also nursing homes in addition to being residential homes. This consisted of patients in various states of being bed-bound and terminally ill, stuck in wheelchairs or beds. This aspect of the care homes horrified my father and he would therefore not consider them as eligible for Judy. There were two possible places that were under consideration. One was a residential care home specializing in Alzheimer's care, and the other was a new care home, with impressive fittings and most bizarrely, a nice carpet throughout that my father was most taken with, and that he insisted my mother would be particularly happy with.

It was discussed with my mother's assigned care worker at the assessment unit, and after speaking with the Manager at the residential home, she was in agreement that the Laxey Glen Care Home, specializing in Alzheimer's care was suitable for my mother's needs. My mother was familiar with the setting as the premises used to be a public house and music venue some years back, when the tourist industry on the island was thriving. My father and mother had frequented the place in their younger days with many happy memories of it. The building itself was surrounded by a beautiful glen with a river meandering through it, with majestic green tall trees. Views of the formal Victorian gardens could be seen from the rear of the property. The rooms were bright and airy with the high ceilings expected in such a period property. The staff were all cheerful and friendly, with the female manager being personable, easy going and empathetic.

We revisited the care home and had some informed discussions with the manager. We could visit whenever we liked and could take my mother out at any time we wished to. There was a hairdresser next-door to the care home, which pleased my father as Judy loved having her hair done. Laxey was a small village which was also halfway between my father's house and our house. The solution, although tough, seemed to make sense. A meeting was arranged at the unit. The Mental Health team had visited Laxey Glen Care Home at some other point in time and had discussed all of Judith's needs and had explained her condition to the manager there. Other residents at the home suffered with dementia too. All agreed that Judith was a suitable candidate for residential care at the unit and that the care home could fulfil Judith's requirements. There was a lift to Judith's room on the third floor and the large window in her bedroom looked over the beautiful glen trees and scenic tiered gardens. We felt happy that Judith could watch the dogs being walked in the glen, and the birds flitting around in the trees. She loved nature and we felt that this secure environment would adequately meet her requirements, whilst providing the beauty and serenity of the natural environment. We could also bring the little dog, Kana, in to see Judith, which was paramount to my mother's pleasure in life. A meeting was then arranged at the assessment unit. It included my father, myself, my husband, the assigned care worker, the Consultant Psychiatrist; a senior mental health worker, plus another mental health nurse, along with Judith herself. The Psychiatrist explained that Judith had an Alzheimer-type dementia and the treatment plan was to continue with all the current medication. None of which was discussed.

On the day of my mother's transfer from the assessment unit to the care home, Judith was very excited. We had collected a few belongings of hers from my parents' bungalow, including photos and pictures that would be familiar to her, and placed them around her room and on her bedside table. Judith was brought to the new care home from the unit, by her care worker Marie. My mother greeted everybody at the home, as if it was her first day at work. She even helped some of the elderly residents into their chairs. We laughed with Judith and she settled in immediately, thriving on all the attention. We all got into the lift which smelled of a canteen as it was next to the kitchen. The doors closed and Judith was giddy and excited as the lift moved slowly upwards. The bell dinged as we reached the floor and Judy imitated that noise like a baby might. We entered her allocated room. It was cold and appeared to have no heating on. Judith was already busy inspecting the room and talking about the photographs that we had placed there already. We turned on the flat screen television and the two female staff brought us all coffee and biscuits. There was a single bed against the back wall, in the middle of the room. It was adequately made-up, but nothing more. Two pillows with stripy blue and cream pillowcases, a fitted sheet to match and a single duvet with a matching cover, that appeared insufficient given the cold temperature. The room had an en-suite toilet, shower and hand basin. It was comfortably furnished with a couple of comfy chairs; a coffee table; a bookshelf; a TV unit with flat screen TV; a couple of bedside units and an over-bed table. From the two huge windows in the room overlooking the garden, one could see the sky and the seagulls soaring high on the thermals, then swooping down suddenly. My mother was entranced by the view. The room was large with thick carpeting. Judith began to dance around in the room with childish enthusiasm, singing to herself as she went. Sometime later when we left, she seemed happy and relaxed. My father appeared comfortable with leaving her there too. They kissed on the lips and hugged goodbye. They told one another that they loved each other. My father promised Judy that he would see her tomorrow. She said goodbye and, "I love you Jim".

The next day, myself, my husband and Kana the Chihuahua, all arranged to make a visit to the care home in the afternoon. On the way there I felt very anxious, dreading seeing my mother in that setting. When we pulled up into the carpark in front of the imposing Victorian building, I immediately noticed my father's car – a pale metallic green Hyundai Matrix – a car that was high to ride in and easy for my father, who was registered disabled with rheumatoid arthritis, to get in and out of. The little dog by this point was all excited, jumping around and panting frantically. She knew that she was going somewhere different and she thrived on seeing new places and new people.

I took her for a brief stroll into the tranquil gardens, in hope that she would not urinate in the care home, not that I thought she would for one moment – but – better safe than sorry. She hurriedly peed and jumped up on my legs, begging for us to show her the big surprise. We climbed up the steep concrete steps to the front of the care home door. I took a piece of paper from my pocket and keyed the numbers written down on it, into the keypad entry system. The door gave a loud clank, at which point I pushed it forward and stepped inside, holding the dog to my chest. There were a few patients in the foyer. All their faces lit up when they saw Kana. They shuffled over with their hands outstretched. The dog grinned from ear to ear and licked the hands that were trying to stroke her, and then some faces, as they got closer to her. There were coos of delight; perhaps a little bit of excitement added to their otherwise routine day.

From the corner of my eye, I could see my mother and father slowly walking towards the lift entrance. My mother spotted us and ran over, shouting, "Oh my Kana". Judy picked her up and hugged her close to her face, planting a big kiss on her fluffy forehead. The dog began licking my mother's face with enthusiasm and mutual affection. Both were overjoyed to see each other. My mother grabbed the hand of another female resident. She was a slim pale lady, with long straight dark and grey hair that was tied into a ponytail. She was still a very elegant lady with a sweet, yet mischievous grin and dark brown eyes. I anticipated that she was probably late seventies or early eighties. My mother on the other hand was just sixty-nine years old, had dark auburn dyed hair; had very youthful, unlined skin; high cheeks bones with full cheeks along with a stocky size sixteen to eighteen frame, and a height of about 5ft 9. The two ladies barged off to the dining room to sit down with Kana, who was in my mother's arms. We all followed them. My mother had the dog on her knee sitting at a round oak dining table. Shirley, my mother's new-found friend, sat next to them. Both ladies petted the dog, who was more than happy with all the attention. My father also pulled up a chair, followed by myself and my husband. A couple of girls who were health care assistants offered us all a coffee or tea and brought some biscuits too. They brought the dog a bowl of water. The dining room was large with a dado rail and a picture rail running around it. The ceilings were high with beautiful chandeliers that adorned the centre. The door to the kitchen was propped open to reveal a full stainless-steel kitchen. Two antique oak sideboards were on either side of the dining room, displaying breakfast cereals in packets; glassware; tea urns; cutlery and condiments. It was a setting reminiscent of a small hotel or guest house. The two ladies were chattering together about the dog, whilst stroking and playing with Kana's long fluffy fur and splayed tail. It was lovely to see two ladies with dementia getting along so well, without a care in the world.

The care home manager, a pale lady with gingerish hair and a kind face, called Karen, came over to speak to my father and me. She explained that Judith had settled in well and was, to be quite honest, under the impression that she worked in the care home, as opposed to being a resident. She had been helping the more elderly residents in and out of their chairs, and had assisted them in moving from room to room. Judith had slept very well; had washed and showered with minimal assistance. At lunchtime she had eaten all her lunch and had taken all her medication when requested. My father and I were so delighted to hear this. We were both racked with guilt over my mother having been placed in the care home and to hear that she was enjoying the environment was of some comfort. Perhaps this was the best decision after all. She had more activities to keep her occupied and more varied company. The frustration and aggression that we had all witnessed from Judy, may have been partly caused by boredom we thought, and perhaps through the frustration that my father had suffered, by trying to cope as best he could too. At the end of each visit, we said our goodbyes to Judith. She always clung on to Jim and gave him a long and often dramatic kiss on the lips, much to the amusement of the other residents. Judith would often laugh and bow, loving the attention.

Christmas 2011 was only weeks away, and we were all aware of how difficult this time of year was going to be. My father had opted to have Christmas lunch in the care home with my mother. The rest of us would visit Judith on Christmas morning.

5

The Cold Wind

Christmas Day arrived, and we drove the six miles to the care home in the morning. We brought some presents for Judith to open. We were all dreading the scenario but put on a brave face and cheery façade. The care home was beautifully decorated with a fine tall Christmas tree in the foyer. Most of the baubles were taken from the tree by various residents and taken back to their room. Judith was indeed one of the biggest culprits and had them stashed on her bedside table.

When we arrived my father's car was already parked up. We went inside the care home and wished everybody a Happy Christmas. Residents were wandering around with paper hats on. Even residents on Zimmer frames were shuffling along with a brightly coloured paper hats on, lopsided at various angles, some wearing garlands of tinsel. The whole place had a lovely jovial feel about it and the residents were mostly cheerful. Some wore Christmas jumpers and others looked like they were wearing new slippers. The home even smelled of Christmas; spicy with a hint of Christmas lunch. We scoured the ground floor for my parents, but they were nowhere to be seen. We took the lift to Judith's room. As soon as we came out of the lift, we came face to face with my father. He was clearly raging. Apparently, Judy was ill. She had indigestion and a sore throat. I told my father I would go back downstairs and ask the staff for some medicine. I found one of the health care assistant girls, wished her Happy Christmas and asked for some medicinal assistance for my mother. The girl explained that she had got Judy ready this morning and informed me that Judith was perfectly well earlier and had eaten breakfast, as well as being in good spirits. She had only taken ill when my father arrived. She claimed that my mother was, "putting it on". She explained that there was nobody on duty, to prescribe the medicine required. I returned to my mother's room and let my father know the circumstances. Judith was lying in bed under the duvet, complaining of a sore throat. Nigel volunteered to go back to our house to fetch some Rennie tablets and some Strepsil throat lozenges. This appeased my father somewhat. He appeared angry with Judith for feeling ill and not wishing to acknowledge Christmas Day, or wish anybody a, 'Happy Christmas'. Judith lay in her bed and complained incessantly about indigestion and a sore throat. We played some Christmas music on the CD player, but this did nothing to brighten her spirits. We opened some cards that we had brought for her and placed them around her room. One of the girls came in and took our drinks order for tea and coffee. Five minutes later she came back with biscuits too. As we chatted and sometimes stopped to sing along with the CD, Judith's spirits began to lift a little and a smile came to her face. My father and I managed to persuade her to get out of bed and open a couple of presents, but she appeared slightly upset about ripping the paper, and became concerned about putting it back together again. By the time that Nigel arrived back with some Strepsils and Rennies, Judith was in an altogether better mood. She agreed to take the medicine anyway, and happily danced with us to some of the Christmas songs playing. It was not dissimilar to entertaining a small kid, making sure that they remained on their best behaviour by keeping them occupied and engaged in activity.

After another hour or so, myself and Nigel left, leaving my father to have lunch at the care home with Judith and the other residents. We returned to finish preparing the lunch that would be attended by my daughter Sophie, her partner Chris; Nigel's brother, Roly, along with his girlfriend.

On the way back to our house, I felt really confused and stressed, even Nigel expressed his concern at how my father was treating my mother. My father seemed to be continually shouting at Judy for losing items – mainly her reading glasses. She had three pairs that he had brought to the Care Home for her. Every visit he would insist on accounting for all three pairs. He would sternly ask Judy where her glasses were, and when she failed to find them, he would go on to explain how much the glasses cost to buy. It appeared to be a continually futile exercise, but each visit would follow the same routine. My father would then go on to inform the care home staff that Judy had lost her glasses, and the staff would swiftly engage a search party to find them – one bright red framed pair; one sky blue framed pair and another pair of gold framed glasses. It was a ritual that caused a continual amount of tension and anxiety to Judith. Since my father's stroke, his patience had clearly worn a little thin. Nigel on the other hand was greatly aggrieved at travelling the journey back to our house to fetch the throat lozenges and indigestion tablets, which, when he had returned, there appeared to be no real requirement for. It was times like these, when Judith's symptoms manifested themselves as almost, "manufactured and staged". It was bewildering and frustrating. We all knew that something very "unfeigned" was occurring in Judith, but it was not a consistent illness – sometimes undeniably dementia-like and at other times a pretence-like condition. Nigel was annoyed at returning with the medication for Judith, but receiving no thanks from my father for having done so, and still no "Happy Christmas", from him. I tried to explain that this Christmas was an unprecedented experience for my parents; the first time they had been separated for it in over forty years, and the saddest Christmas for my father, ever. That, on top of his residual stroke attributes, explained his lack of consideration.

Back at our house, we busied around; cooking; tidying; preparing; laying the table; playing Christmas music and turning the Christmas tree lights on – all in an attempt to replicate some sort of festive normality. I, on the other hand, wished that I could just sit in a darkened cupboard, alone and still; to address my feelings, as opposed to suppressing them.

An hour or so later, the dog, Kana, started barking and rushing into the kitchen to see us, before promptly dashing back to the lounge. This was a sure sign of visitors. Nigel's brother and his girlfriend arrived onto the driveway in her bright red Audi. We all exchanged our Christmas greetings, hugs and kisses, then indulged in a glass of champagne each. It WAS past midday and it WAS Christmas. Some minutes later, Sophie and Chris arrived in their maroon VW campervan, accompanied by the canine choral rejoice from Kana. This was followed by more festive pleasantries and another glass of champagne each. Sophie and Chris had visited the care home, before arriving at our house, to see her grandparents. They hadn't stayed too long, as there was some conflict between her grandparents and some other residents, over the seating arrangements in the lounge. Sophie and Chris did not expand any further on the situation in any detail.

As was our usual tradition at Christmas, we all exchanged gifts and chatted, updating each other on life events. We also put on the singing and dancing five cuddly reindeers, that the dog was customarily overjoyed at attacking and wrestling to the floor, one by one. I flitted between cooking, chatting and preparing for lunch. Sophie and Roly chatted with me in the kitchen. Nigel kept the champagne flowing – I stopped after my second glass. Alcohol, cooking and serving I considered to be a bad combination. My organisational skills were laboured at the best of times. The table looked fabulous with a beautiful white linen Christmas tablecloth with a contrasting red velvet runner; silver napkin rings, with white linen napkins. Two bottles of wine; one New Zealand Marlborough Sauvignon Blanc and one good Spanish Rioja. A starter of fresh broccoli and stilton soup, with warm, crusty, (exploding), bread rolls. Lunch consisted of a combination of turkey and gammon; chestnut stuffing, brussel sprouts; cranberries, roast chestnuts, roast potatoes; cheesy mash potatoes; peas; Yorkshire puddings; bread sauce; carrot and swede mash, and .... The vegetarian turkey – nut roast served with a rich mushroom sauce. All served with two big jugs of homemade gravy. The dog got stuck into her Christmas lunch too, while we indulged in the colossal platefuls of food. Out of our guests, Roly, who is a big frame of a man, would win the 'Biggest Eater Award', and Chris,' The Fastest Eater Award'; he was a purposeful eater. We all chatted, pulled crackers, told jokes, wore silly paper hats, supped wine and leisurely cleared our plates of any trace of Christmas lunch. Although Roly would leave his brussel sprouts, I always put them on his plate for a joke, knowing full well that he hated them. I would normally slip them under some potatoes, or under the Yorkshire pudding. He would roar with laughter when he discovered their presence.

We all then retired into the lounge to allow our lunch to digest for a little while, before further partaking in some Christmas pudding, brandy cream and fresh cream too.

I was struggling with the festive spirit. Agreeably two glasses of champagne and a glass of Rioja had lessened my anxiety over my mother and father, but I still felt flat; numb; dead inside of my body. No joy; no pleasure – just empty. I still had an overwhelming desire to hide in the cupboard under the stairs. To be still with my thoughts. Undisturbed and alone. To think; to analyse; to evaluate. To cry; to shout; to sleep – to wake-up and to realise that it was all a horrible nightmare.

The Christmas pudding was now cooked. We all ate while talking and discussing various topics, namely work and family. Thankfully, the conversation flowed effortlessly. I was putting on a brave face, trying to relax and be jovial; not wanting to put a dampener on anybody's Christmas Day. After coffee and chocolates, Roly left later that afternoon, taking his bagful of presents with him. No sooner had we all settled back into the lounge chatting, when Kana the dog started barking, followed by a car that pulled onto the driveway. It was my father's green-coloured Hyundai Matrix. Amazingly, he had my mother with him in the passenger seat. We were all a little taken aback by this. After my father's stroke, he was struggling to walk; he was unsteady on his feet and was still dragging his left foot somewhat. The steep steps from the Victorian Care Home were very difficult for him to manage and he clung to the handrails when climbing down. Judith on the other hand was fit and physically healthy, and very strong-willed. Yet, despite this, she still needed prompting and directing.

Nigel went to the front door and welcomed them in. On entering the lounge, we all wished each other 'Happy Christmas'. Judith's eyes lit up when she saw her granddaughter, and Sophie's partner. Judith immediately remarked, 'Chris, how lovely to see you. Thank you for coming'. The silence that followed, told the story. We were utterly flabbergasted that Judith had remembered his name. The last time that she had encountered him was exactly one year previous. How on earth could she recall his name, yet finding her way to the bathroom was problematic. We were all stunned. How could this be? What on earth was going on with Judith? The conversation with her quickly declined into jumbled sentences, jumping from topic to topic, forgetting the thread of the conversation without any cohesion. We were all clearly uncomfortable seeing her so confused, random and jumbled with her speech. She was forgetting what she wanted to say mid-sentence, but instead of being frustrated, or angry with herself, Judith found it highly amusing and was laughing enthusiastically. We all attempted to laugh with her and reassure her. We offered chocolates to everybody. Judith was infant-like, snatching the box when offered to her, quickly stuffing two into her mouth at time, bulging at the cheeks like a little hamster, and then she guarded the box with her life, grinning manically and attempting a chocolate-stifled laugh. My father insisted upon removing the sweets from her possession, explaining that she would make herself sick. Reluctantly, she handed the treasure over, but her drooping bottom lip said it all. We all laughed and she revelled in the attention. She had reverted to being an infant – a cheeky, mischievous girl, with a captivating naughty smile, along with a twinkle of disobedience in her eyes. My father noticed her unsettling nature, and promptly advised that he had best return with her to the care home. Judith clearly had no recollection of where she was going back to, as she willingly hugged and kissed us. She exclaimed what a wonderful day she'd had, then happily followed Jim out to the car, and got in unaided and without any hint of resistance. I asked my father to ring as soon as he got back home safely, after returning Judith.

Later that night, at around 9pm, my father rang. He explained that he had immense trouble leaving Judy in the care home. She had been shouting and screaming at him. She had banged on the windows of the care home and when he had gotten outside, she banged on them so hard that he thought that she would break them. I could hear in his voice that he was near to tears, whilst recounting the events. I asked him if he wanted to stay at our house, but he declined the offer, saying that he wanted to be alone, then changing his stance and saying that he wished to be with Judy. He sounded exhausted, saying that he wished that he was dead, as he was no longer any use to her. I reminded him of how much she adored to see him, and how she was so fortunate to have such a caring husband. He began sobbing down the telephone, saying that he wanted Judith home, but acknowledging that he just could not cope with her. I informed him that everybody knew that, as I myself could not cope either. Perhaps his unnecessary guilt abated, and we said our goodnights to each other. I placed the telephone receiver down and tears began streaming down my face. Such a cruel situation; out of everybody's control.

6
The Changing Wind

Perhaps with a little haste, I had booked a short one-week holiday away to the Gambia with Nigel. Normally, at that time of year we would take our annual holiday to South Goa, but perhaps this year it was not possible. Yet this was only one week away, and at the time of booking, everything appeared stable with both my mother's and father's situation. Both myself and Nigel had been ill for most of the week in Gambia, with a heavy cold. We had not really enjoyed the holiday at all. Therefore, on returning from this holiday, and seeing everything seemed stable with my mother, we felt safe enough to book three weeks to South Goa, at the end of February, to catch up with friends there, that we met up with annually. Judith seemed well settled and my father seemed well too.

Not so long into the new year, the manageress at the care home explained that they could not cope with Judith's behaviour. She wandered constantly at night, entering other residents' rooms and frightening them. Often, she was disturbed and getting frustrated or upset. The manageress, Karen, told us that despite Diazepam – enough to knock a horse out, she informed us – it wasn't touching Judith, and she was still taking her Chloral Betaine 707mg tablet too. Karen had also asked Judith's G.P. to visit her. The G.P. in-turn wrote a letter asking for help from the Mental Health Services and asking for a review of her medication. The letter was dated 02 February 2012 to the Older Persons Mental Health Services.

Part of this letter read:-

“This lady is very labile in her mood and agitation levels. She has been persistently very down and tearful since arriving at Glen House, and we did try a small 10mg Citalopram dose, but she quickly became even more agitated with this and it was stopped. My partner introduced a small dose of diazepam prior to her spouse’s visits, but this proved of limited benefit. We would greatly appreciate any advice you could offer us on Mrs Allen“.

The reply from the Mental Health Services was dated 06 February 2012. The latter part of this letter informed the G.P. that, ‘I do feel that changes in medication may not always have a therapeutic effect. I have discussed current concerns with Dr. Jagus and he will be maintaining an on-going review of her medication.

I have regular contact with staff at Glen House and they do appear to be managing Mrs Allen well, despite the difficulties that have arisen.

I hope this has offered some form of help//advice regarding this lady’s health care requirements that will enable her to reach her optimum level of functioning’.

Incidentally, Dr. Jagus’ review of medication, without assessing the patient, was to increase her Pregablin script from 50mg once daily, to 50mg twice daily. No further help was offered to either the G.P. or the Care Home.

It may have been as a direct result of no forthcoming help or advice from Mental Health Services, that sometime in the middle of February, Karen explained to my father that Judith would have to move to another establishment. It was suggested that she needed a Nursing Home, not because she was in anyway physically impaired, but because they felt Judith would benefit and thrive in a one-to-one environment, and required that level of attention to get showered and dressed, due to her refusal and agitation levels. Judith’s mood swings were severe at times and could range from being subdued and calm to be near hysterical and aggressive. Her and another dementia patient had, at some point, had an altercation which resulted in Judith having bite marks on her arms and the other lady having bruises. The incident was not witnessed by staff members.

My father rang me in the afternoon to inform me that the care home was, 'evicting', Judith, and that the Mental Health Services had told him this. Understandably, he was angered and upset, which in-turn annoyed me. My father had suffered a stroke and was not to be subjected to undue stress. I immediately rang the Mental Health Services who casually informed me that Judith did not need to move straight away; only when we had found a suitable alternative for her. I was livid. Moreover, my poor mother had been assessed at the unit for some three weeks and we were assured that they felt Glen House was appropriate for her needs. Yet, less than three months later, everybody concerned is stating that it is now unsuitable for her, and that this establishment does not have the experience or staffing levels to deal with her.

The timing of this decision was unfortunate for myself and my husband. We had decided to take the plunge and had booked the Goa holiday for three weeks on 28 February. Things had seemed stable enough to go, but obviously the change of care homes would most likely happen whilst we were away.

I had shamefully advised my Mother's Care Worker, Marie, that with the most unfortunate timing, myself and my husband had a holiday planned to Goa. We had booked our flights at a time when my mother was very well settled at the Care Home, and that there was no way of knowing that the situation would indeed change so quickly. She did appear to sympathise with the issue and was kind enough to inform us that she would help with moving my mother to new premises. Judith would now require a nursing home, as explained, not because of any mobility issues, but due to the requirement of the one-to-one care that the professionals felt that Judith required. To keep her occupied and engaged in activities; to assist her with showering and her day-to-day routine, and more importantly to assist with her volatile mood swings, using distraction tactics. My father and I once again paid visit to numerous nursing homes, but due to his lack of mobility, he wished for Judith to be in his hometown of Ramsey. He eventually took the decision to move her to Beaconsfield Nursing Home. They had recently opened a new EMI (Elderly Mentally Infirm), unit there. It was spanking brand new and looked suitably impressive, with a pretty garden and a lounge overlooking this. Her bedroom was beautifully appointed with freshly painted bright décor and stylish furniture. Judith would be their first in-patient to the unit. Marie would ensure the move for Judith was smooth, and she would assist my father in any way that she could. I felt immensely relieved to hear this, although the guilt of not being there for the move, and indeed out of the country, was far greater. I knew that I was letting my father down, by not being around to support him, but I also knew that Nigel was bearing the brunt of my parents' health issues, and he deserved to have some quality time too. Together, was what we desperately needed. To try and rebuild on any foundations that remained.

Leaving my father with my mother's moving of care homes, was particularly difficult, but he insisted that we still went to Goa, and he was adamant that he would be perfectly fine. He was even looking forward to visiting Judith in her new place. The driving would take him maybe five minutes only. Marie would be there for him and support him too in any way.

After leaving the island and reaching London, my pure sense of freedom kicked in. Selfishly, like leaving a nightmare and returning into the real world. The guilt remained, but it was overridden by the sheer beauty of being free.

Goa is everything I had ever dreamed of. The South of Goa is rustic and charming. Engulfed by swaying coconut palms, pale sand and beautiful blue seas. The greenery is spectacular, and the natural wildlife is astounding. Birds everywhere; kingfishers; kites; eagles; bulbuls with their sweet song; Indian rollers. The list was endless. Wild pigs darting around; lazy cows meandering around; shiny black water buffalo wallowing in deep pools, with lotus leaves hanging from the heads, like dreadlocks. Goa is where nature soothes the soul and where beach dogs are overjoyed to see you. Never a minute without some part of nature surprising you. My heart will forever be in South Goa with its beautiful rivers, stunning beaches and deserted coves. Playful dolphins in the ocean and cheeky monkeys scampering across roads and clambering in trees. For me it was heaven. Romantically where all your troubles float away, if only for three weeks. The hotel where we were staying was family run and rural. The small balcony overlooked paddy fields where the mist hung over them early in the morning, lifting as the morning sun arose. Playful dogs could be seen chasing the pigs, who squealed with excitement, as the morning awakened. Squeaking stripy squirrels launched through the palm trees and eagles soared above in the perfect blue sky. A pure antidote to any stress.

We remained in daily contact with my father and he updated us on occurring events. I could hear his voice crack a couple of times when talking with him. He was struggling emotionally, and I was wracked with guilt. I just wanted to hug him. Yet, it wasn't until two days before we came back from Goa, that Judy moved from Laxey Glen House to Beaconsfield Nursing Home in Ramsey.

The move went smoothly, and father informed us that Judith was enjoying the environment and the garden especially. They had taken tea and biscuits together in the garden and the weather had been pleasant. All her belongings had accompanied her, and she was in fact the only resident on that floor, at that present time. My father was less than happy with the nursing home fees of nearly £3,500 per month, but as he realised, there were no other options available. He sadly could not look after her; he was struggling with his own mobility. Her labile moods, hallucinations, night-time roaming and psychotic episodes required professional attention.

7

The Stillness Arrives

I knew once we had landed back at Ronaldsway Airport, in the Isle of Man, that I would visit my mother and father as soon as possible, which would probably be in the afternoon later that day. Travelling back from the airport seemed dull and grey. The tress looked stark and the sky moody and threatening. My heart ached to see the swaying palm trees of Goa again, and the vivid, alive greenery of that landscape. Back on the island I suddenly felt my energies drain and the burden of negativity return. What was lying in store for us all, as a family?

Travelling over the mountain road later that day, from Onchan on the East coast, to Ramsey on the North coast, was sometimes a beautiful journey, but that day it seemed grim. The mountains appeared lifeless, without any trees; the terrain stark. I needed to snap-out quickly from my mood, and stop being selfish. A beautiful tropical holiday followed by gloom. Back to the start again.

We pulled up into the carpark at Beaconsfield Nursing Home, and we were pleasantly surprised to see my father's car was already in situ. In the bright clear reception area inside of the building, a cheery lady of Zambian origin, (she informed us), greeted me and Nigel, and gladly filled us in about Judith's arrival there two days ago, and on her progress. So far, my father and mother had eaten their lunch together on both days, and "Jim and Judy", seemed happy with the new placement. She led us into a lift, which took us up to the third floor. The décor and furnishings were impressive, and as we went through the double French doors, I could see my father and mother sitting and holding hands, in the bright spacious lounge. Tea, coffee and biscuits adorned the coffee table before them. My mother's eyes lit-up with joy when she spotted Nigel and me. She rushed over to hug us like an excited infant, beaming from ear to ear. My father in contrast looked deathly pale and grey in the face. He hugged us both, but it seemed that all was not well with him. A slight lady in her 50's with a weather-beaten face, came and introduced herself, as Judy's carer; she brought Nigel a cup of coffee, and me a mug of tea, accompanied by biscuits. She then asked if we minded if she went for a cigarette, seeing as we were all with Judith. It appeared a little unprofessional, but we agreed that she could. Judith galloped around showing me her room and the items that were in it. She dragged me by the hand into the bathroom, eagerly showing me the shower. We then went into the lounge and then into the dining kitchen. She was full of the joys of spring. Perhaps this was the best place for my mother to settle. She certainly appeared happy. Later, the carer explained that Judith seemed to be under the impression that the whole unit of the floor was her new house. She was delighted with it, but had repeatedly asked the carer who she was, and why she was in Judith's house. We laughed as the carer relayed this too us, but I could see that the cracks were forming.

My parents wedding anniversary was looming. They had been married for forty-eight years. Judith's sister, sister-in-law and brother were coming over to visit from the UK. They were all aware of the current situation, but I pre-empted that the reality of it would be harder than they realised. Judith particularly loved her younger brother and was very excited at the prospect of him visiting. The family members were staying at our house for the duration. We always had great times, and I hoped this time would be no different.

They arrived on 20 March 2012, and the weather was unusually sunny and warm.

The next day following their arrival, we went to visit Judith. As we all arrived on the third floor of the unit, the lift doors opened and we could see Jim and Judy sitting together as normal, holding hands. Judy's brother, Bryan, spoke first, "Hello Judy". She turned and shot out of her chair at speed, with pure innocent excitement, running over to him and throwing her arms around him. This was followed by floods of tears. She hugged each one of us in turn, whilst still crying. They were tears of elation; she was overwhelmed. We all sat around in the comfortable chesterfield-style leather chairs, and tea, coffee, biscuits and cakes were brought to us by the care worker. Judy could not stop talking, jumping from topic to topic. Some rambles were comprehensible, some left us completely lost. Sometimes Judith laughed and at other times she became irritated by her lack of cohesion in her sentences. Her sister-in-law, Cherie, suggested playing some CD's on the music system. (Cherie had been working with older patients for a large part of her working career and was very adept at dealing with similar scenarios). Judith was overjoyed and started dancing around, as if in some jazzy nightclub, dragging each one of us by the hands to join her. We were all in the lounge and all dancing to Abba songs. Judith lavished in the attention and began exercising too, bending to touch her toes. We were all shocked by her flexibility. Even Cherie commented, "What happened to Judy's bad back?". Judith had suffered with back pain for many years and had undergone one back operation. There was obviously not one iota of back pain now.

Bryan had thoughtfully brought a photograph album, compiled of family photos from years ago. He had read that it was helpful for dementia patients to have such an item. He sat with Judith reminiscing about old times. Judith looked on, beaming whole-heartedly, from ear to ear. She sighed and asked Cherie to make us gin and tonics. We all burst out laughing, and Judy roared with laughter too.

When it was time for us to leave, Judith became agitated and tried to come down in the lift with us. The care worker came to our aid by attempting to distract Judith, but by this point, my mother was most perplexed as to why her, "little brother", was leaving without her. My father remained behind with my mother, but this was of no consolation to Judy at all. We speedily left at the first opportunity, leaving my father and the care-worker to deal with the aftermath of our leaving. We had explained to Judith that we would be meeting up the next day at Peel beach for a stroll on the beach with Kana the dog, and to have an ice cream there too.

Later that night, after returning to our house, we all became nostalgic, talking about family times, when Judy was well. Bryan, Judy's brother, Cherie her sister-in-law and Ruth her sister, were all shocked by my father's appearance, and his newly acquired insensitivity to Judy's condition, following his last stroke. He looked so frail, drawn and grey in the face. We all agreed that Judy had been feisty all of her life, (a characteristic that made her formidable as a County Councillor in her prior town of Newport, in Shropshire), but at the same time she could reign-it-in, when needed. Yet now, with the dementia, it was impossible for her to control such traits. This was proving to be the most difficult aspect in dealing with Judith in her condition now.

That evening was cold. Too cold to sit out in the garden, that was illuminated by an array of lights and a superbly lit-up rockery and pond area, so we sat in the conservatory, overlooking the gardens and had a meal accompanied by drinks, whilst reminiscing about good times together.

The following morning we all got up to the joys of another unusually sunny day for March. We sat in the rustic beamed kitchen and enjoyed a hearty full English breakfast. Bryan, despite the fact that he was suffering with inoperable secondary breast cancer, was in good spirits, and he and Nigel undertook the washing-up, whilst Cherie, Ruth and I took Kana, the dog for a walk down to the glen, following the gurgling stream on our route. When we returned, we all had a coffee, before heading off in our car, with Kana, for our day out to Peel.

Peel had one large sandy bay, and one smaller cove; both were complemented and adjoined to the impressive Peel Castle, and a picturesque harbour and marina, where seals could be seen, peeking curiously out of the sea. Peel was an oldie-worldie place, which was especially pretty on a sunny day, when the sun sparkled in the clear blue waters, surrounded by powdery pale sand. We passed by the boats moored in the marina, bobbing up and down on the still water.

Boats of all different shapes and sizes. Some tall, elegant teak yachts, down to the 5hp outboard motor dinghies. Some people were cleaning their boats, others were sailing them in or out of the harbour, and some more extravagant people were sipping wine onboard of theirs, but still moored up. Enjoying the life. Seagulls were soaring high in the sky, whilst others were perched on masts, screeching their hearty calls, with their heads upturned to the sky, appearing in full praise of the day. Ducks paddled by in search of generous passers-by with a bag of bread.

When we arrived in the car park at the little sandy cove of Fenella beach, my father was parked up with my mother in the passenger seat. My father spotted us first, then Judith hurriedly alighted the car, rushing over to greet us in haste, ignorant of any traffic that may have been passing. We all stood in anticipation, but Judith ignored us all and made a bee-line for Kana, snatching her up in her arms from Cherie, with an accusingly stern look on her face. The dog rejoiced, licking Judith all over her face; my mother euphoric to see the dog. My father followed on, and we hugged him in turn. My mother didn't notice us, and was all consumed by Kana, whom she had already started walking with towards the beach. We all laughed and followed on behind them. The beach was relatively quiet considering it was a warm, blue sky day. We sat as a group on the low sea wall, watching in amusement as Kana chased a ball that we took in turns to repeatedly throw. It was a small tennis-type ball, golf-ball sized and adored by the slightly larger-than-normal Chihuahua. Bryan and Nigel strolled off to fetch some ice cream. On their return with the small individual tubs with spoons, Kana instantly fell out of love with her game of ball. She was now firmly fixated with the ice cream that Judith then proceeded to feed to Kana, by means of her finger. The dog was delighted, and my mother was beaming with joy too. We all sat for about a further hour, basking in the sunshine and watching the goings-on of the beach, before Judith started to lose concentration and started to become agitated, rummaging manically through her handbag, as if looking for something of notable importance. We all then gathered our belongings; Cherie picked up Kana and we headed towards the cars. My mother's walking was a little slow as she shuffled up the boat ramp and towards the vehicles. When Judith arrived at the car, she said sternly to Cherie, "Give me Kana. You are not keeping her". Cherie gently went to hand over Kana, who, low in mid-air, scrambled and jumped to the floor, unperturbed. Judith rushed down to pick her up, whilst exclaiming, "Oh my God", in a panicked manner. She looked at Cherie while biting her bottom lip with her top teeth, in an angry, almost threatening manner. Judith then stormed off to the passenger seat of my father's car, got into the car with the dog on her lap, whilst seething, with the sullen face of a spoiled child. I went over to her, opened the door and gave her a hug. I persuaded her to hand Kana over to me, as I explained that she needed a little walk to allow her to do her business. Unhappy, but relenting, my mother surrendered the dog to me. I then walked Kana to the beach and out of Judith's sight, as soon as possible. Once my father's car was out of sight, we re-grouped and walked around the castle to look for seals. We found them and Kana frenzily barked on spotting them. We laughed at the pluckiness of such a small dog.

8

The Calm Before the Storm

The following day was my parents' anniversary; 23 March 2012. It was their forty nineth Wedding Anniversary. Once again, we had asked the Care Home for their permission to take Judith out. They had eagerly permitted that. We had planned on going out for a celebratory meal, not so far from Ramsey, to a small country pub, The Grosvenor, in a village called Andreas. It was a quaint traditional pub on the edge of the village. It was once one of Judy and Jim's favourite places to eat. We were meeting my mother and father at the Care Home, and would proceed to the white-washed pub, after presenting them both with their anniversary cards and gifts. When we arrived at the third floor of the unit, Jim and Judy were sitting holding hands as usual, in the lounge. They didn't notice us arrive this time, but they were both pleased to see us. The care worker had helped Judith, dress smartly in beige linen trousers; a cream blouse and a dusky pink cardigan. Her now-greying hair had been neatly brushed and she was wearing a lick of pale lipstick. We all told her how lovely she looked, and Judith seemed to beam with pride. She looked at Jim, told him that she loved him and leaned into him, planting a long, lingering kiss on his mouth. Jim replied, "I love you too Judles", (his pet name for her). His eyes glistened with emotion. We gave Judith the cards and small gifts of chocolates. She hurriedly ripped open the cards and immediately passed them to Jim, without glancing inside of them. She then proceeded to open the chocolates, took two out, promptly stuffed them into her mouth and shoved the box at Jim. She was reminiscent of a kid who had forgotten their manners in all the excitement. We laughed and Jim told her not to eat anymore, as she would not eat her lunch. In defiance, she grabbed the box back and took two more and repeatedly forced them into her already full mouth. We laughed; she laughed a chocolaty laugh, and chocolate shot out of her mouth on to the floor. Judith doubled over with hysterical laughter. My father exclaimed, "Judith", in a stern manner. He was not impressed at his once elegant wife. We all sniggered at her silliness. On regaining her composure, we all headed for the lift and out to the cars in the car park. Judith was so full of life and enthusiasm that day.

When we arrived at the pub, we were led to a reserved table for seven people. We began to order our drinks, but Judy was a little confused. We had to read out her options, then she decided on Coke. We were given the menus to look at and choose our dishes. My father read out the options to Judith again, but she struggled to decide; my father helped her to choose vegetable lasagne. She had been vegetarian for many years now, but sometimes she would forget now and succumb to a bacon sandwich. We chatted over drinks. Sometimes Judith could keep up with the conversation, but at other times struggled and would interrupt with something totally random, and would often lose her train of thought, rambling from one topic to another. Yet Judith was in her element and appeared very happy and reasonably coherent. The meals came and we all enjoyed them. Judith ate most of her food and was eager to have chocolate cake. She was goading us all to have chocolate cake too. Her spirits were high. She even managed to laugh and converse with the landlord of the pub. Together we all had a lovely time and my father appeared very happy, especially with Judith coping so well. We wished them both a very happy anniversary and raised our glasses to them. Judith raised hers too and gave Jim another big kiss on the mouth. After the chocolate cake, which Judith devoured in a matter of minutes, we settled the bill and got up to leave. Nigel and I walked out ahead. As we left, we spotted a friend of ours, with another couple of ladies and stopped for a brief chat. Judith came from behind and said, "Hello", to them. She then told our friend, "They all think I am mental, but I am not". Our friend said, "I don't know about you, but I am". Judith roared with laughter and then said, "Goodbye", to her. No issues with Judith's manner, speech or appropriateness. No outwardly obvious signs of her dementia on that day. The affliction of dementia appeared to be unbelievably inconsistent. We said our "Goodbyes" in the carpark and my father took Judith back to the Nursing Home and settled her back in, sitting in the lounge with her, taking coffee and biscuits. Leaving her alone again, was very difficult for my father, along with her reluctance to allow him to leave. He was suffering immensely with sadness and guilt, in a situation that had no apparent easing in sight.

Bryan, Cherie and Ruth had just one more day left on the island. The weather was fantastic again; we were blessed with so much sunshine for March. Their final day on the island was spent in Laxey; a small coastal village on the East coast. It had a delightful curved bay, surrounded by two headlands and had a picturesque harbour with a small promenade leading from it. The beach had small boulders and stones at the promenade wall and sloped down to a sandy beach when the tide was out, exposing rock pools where children played in search of crabs hiding under seaweed, with their buckets and spades. The light breeze carried the distinct salty smell of the sea. In the upper village was a monumental water wheel, built in the Victorian times, majestically painted in red, black and white, providing views over the green landscape and out to the twinkling blue sea. A photographer's dream. The walk to the top of the wheel was challenging for those in fear of heights, but the panorama provided a just reward.

We lunched in a quaint Mill House restaurant overlooking the river, and a small water wheel turning with the running water. We managed to sit outside in the cobbled courtyard, and enjoyed the sheltered sun, whilst eating our lunch. While we were sitting and eating, my mobile phone rang. It was my father. He explained that we had better not come and see Judy, (as we had planned to), as she was in a particularly difficult mood and very argumentative. The care worker at the unit was finding her behaviour challenging and had rang my father to come and sit with her, in an attempt to raise her spirits. He told me that he would have lunch at the unit with Judy and would then leave and take some rest. I informed him that we would come later and visit him at his bungalow, with Bryan, Cherie and Ruth, but he went on to explain that he'd rather we didn't visit, as he was feeling very exhausted. We said our farewells and I let him know that I would call him later, after his rest. I relayed the conversation to the family, and they agreed it was best not to visit Judy or Jim that day. Judy's brother, Bryan felt a mixture of relief and sadness. On one-hand, he didn't wish to see her in that condition; it saddened him greatly, but on the other-hand, having cancer himself, the future held no certainties for him, and he was therefore concerned about seeing Judy again. Luckily, he had seen her in great spirits the previous day, with lots of happy photographs to show for it.

The next morning Bryan, Cherie and Ruth had an early morning flight to Birmingham airport from the island. We all hugged and kissed, saying our goodbyes. It was emotional, especially for Bryan with his health implications and we all shed a tear without saying too much. After they left, life went on very much as before. Jim was visiting Judith every day for a few hours, and myself and Nigel visited four or five times a week.

The Care Home still had only Judith on their third floor of the unit. They had attempted to integrate her with other patients on the second floor, but Judith proved difficult, argumentative and a little aggressive in her manner with them. She was still under the impression that the third floor of the unit was her, individual new house. Every time Jim visited, she would express her utmost love for him and when he wasn't there, she would be continuously asking for him; at times, shouting for him. On a couple of times, the care worker expressed to me that my mother was a "bully", and that she had never dealt with a case of dementia like hers before. She told me that Judith was a most difficult patient with volatile mood swings. One-minute quiet and calm, but then in a split second that would all change. Judith was experiencing hallucinations at times too, talking to imaginary people and animals, and needed to be constantly attached to her teddy bear. The care worker explained that one of her colleagues who had also dealt with Judith, had signed-off sick, and was refusing to work with Judith again. My father, who was still struggling with his own health and mobility, had been telephoned in the evening on a few occasions, requesting him to come into the unit to assist in calming Judith down, as she would be regularly crying and shouting for him. On numerous times, we were told, that Judith had informed staff of her wish to kill herself. This information was also passed on to Marie and to Judith's Psychiatrist, Dr Jagus. My father explained his frustration to me. He was paying nearly £3,500 per month for Judith to be professionally cared for, as he could not do so, yet he was being called in, at the end of the day, when he was at his most tired. I let the Unit Manager know of my concerns and relayed the same information to Marie, who still visited Judith. She also insisted that Jim should not be subjected to such stress following his stroke. She was very concerned to hear that this was happening and informed me that she would discuss it with the Private Care Home too.

For a few weeks the situation never arose again. Then, as abruptly as it had stopped, it started once more. Only, on those further occasions, Judith almost refused to allow Jim to leave, and staff intervention was needed to distract Judith, whilst Jim made his get-away.

9

The Storm Approaches

One morning, I had a telephone call from my father explaining that he had been called in to the unit to assist with Judith. She had threatened staff with a torrent of abuse and was very threatening in her nature, attempting to break doors and windows. She had attempted to lash out at the care worker too. The previous professional involved with my mother, from the mental health unit had been contacted by Beaconsfield Nursing Home, and a decision had been made to "Section", Judith under the Mental Health Act, Section 2. Two doctors, one of whom would be a Psychiatrist, would have to be present with Judith to ensure the correct protocol was followed. Judith would then be transported by ambulance with police presence, to take her back to the Government EMI unit, Grainagh Court, where she had previously been, prior to her first care home placement. I told my father that I would leave from my house immediately, and I would arrive there shortly. Marie explained that Jim was in a hostage-like situation, with Judith not allowing him to leave his chair in the lounge. Nigel decided to drive over to Ramsey with me, thankfully. My heart was racing, and my legs were trembling with panic. My throat was tightening so much on the way over to Ramsey. I had to calm myself with measured breathing. Never in my life had I experienced such panic and anxiety. I could only imagine how much stress my poor father was under. I prayed he would not suffer another stroke. Please God, take pity on him.

We arrived in the car park. As normal my father's car was there. I had no idea what to expect from the situation, but there was no sign of chaos in the car park. As Nigel and I entered the care home reception, the Care Home Manager appeared, as if waiting for us. He seemed agitated. He began explaining the events of the morning and how Judith had been running up and down the unit, screaming and shouting, banging on windows and doors, swearing and cursing. He also informed me that I was at the centre of her anger, and that she was blaming me for everything and anything. He explained that the unit did not have the facilities to meet Judith's requirements. Previously another member of staff had informed my father that the staff were not trained enough to deal with Judith. Both statements were starting to ring very true. The previous assessment at the mental health unit had proved futile. Clearly another assessment was needed. He went onto explain that Judith would be "Sectioned" but stated that this procedure could take forever and that, "we may be here all night waiting for them to get their act together – they don't rush these things". I was a little taken aback. Was he irritated by the turn of events, or was he talking from experience?". The "us", and "them", seemed a little cutting too. We took the lift to the third-floor unit and were met by the care worker, who began explaining that I wasn't Judith's favourite person today, and that she had been blaming "Victoria", for everything. We entered the unit as normal through the French doors. When my mother spotted us, she came running towards us with a picture in her hands. Upon seeing me she attempted to hit me in the face with it and kick me. Nigel stepped forward as she did so, to intervene and grabbed Judith by both wrists, with much force. She spat in his face, but was looking at me, screaming, "You fucking bitch. All of this is your doing. You fucking little witch". Her green eyes were filled with rage and pure hatred. She looked like she could kill me in an instant. I was so shocked, and immediately retreated into the kitchen, where the care worker shut the door and responded by saying, "Judy has been like this all morning, saying that she hated Victoria. She also said that she wished to kill herself too".

A huge wave of guilt washed over me. Tears were rolling down my cheeks and I was aware that my chin and mouth were quivering uncontrollably. Yet I was questioning the series of events over that past few months. Did my mother actually remember that it was me who had first placed her in the unit? Seriously, could she remember that? It occurred to me that she did in fact recall this event. More staff entered the kitchen. They were all telling me not to enter Judith's unit again, as she was liable to try attacking me again. I was told to go and wait downstairs on the ground floor. I willingly left, but as I entered the lift, I could see the frail figure of my father, hunched over in the chair; his walking stick propped up against the chair. Judith was manically pacing up and down, in front of him. She spotted me and came hurtling towards the French door, grabbing the handle, but thankfully the staff had locked the doors. Judith was frantically banging the doors. Her face grotesquely contorted as she spat abuse towards me.

Once out in the car park, I attempted to regain some composure, or at least stop myself from shaking, when Marie came over. She was disturbingly calm and jovial, explaining that she would go and sit with Judy and Jim, as she believed that she could manage to placate Judith, as she trusted Marie. Nigel came out as Marie passed. She told him that Judith's behaviour was demented, which related directly to her dementia. She was laughing as she spoke. I wanted to ask her which part of this situation was even slightly amusing, but I relented. All of this confused me. It was like a nightmare that I wished I could wake up from.

Shortly afterwards the ambulance arrived. There were discussions for some time amongst the professionals. The two doctors had not arrived, and it would appear that the ambulance crew were refusing to take Judith for fear over their own safety. Talks between them seemed to take ages. The police also arrived. Nigel and I had no idea what was going on, but eventually the ambulance left, without Judith. The police departed too. The unit manager came out, stating again that we would be here all night, sighing with irritation. I was worried for my father. He had now been with Judith for nearly five hours. I found myself praying he would not suffer another stroke.

By now, neither Nigel nor myself had eaten since the night before. My legs were trembling and weak. I suggested grabbing something to eat and drink, as it may be some considerable time until my mother was transferred back to Grainagh Court Mental Health Unit. Marie had asked staff to prepare food for Jim and Judy, and she would sit with them.

Nigel and I drove into Ramsey town and picked up a couple of sandwiches from the Co-op store. We then decided to go to my parents' bungalow and make a coffee and eat our sandwiches. Although I felt sick to the very pit of my stomach, I needed to eat something. The weather was damp and cold. I could not refrain from shivering. My parents' house was dark and grim inside. Still all the blinds and curtains were drawn. The air was dank and musty. My father's distress and depression could be felt in every room. The black and gold fireplace was the only comfort, right next to his electric reclining chair, which had once eased him up from sitting down, due to his rheumatoid arthritis. This illness had forced him into early retirement from his job as a superintendent radiographer, on health grounds, when Jim was in his mid-forties. I remembered well, his swollen twisted fingers and his contorted hideous toes and feet, that he could barely walk upon. My mother had been due to be the next Mayoress of Newport, but she had forgone the prospect due to Jim's health issues. All these memories came flooding back. For a moment, I had forgotten the grim reality of the surreal situation of present. I was deeply disturbed at the chain of events. I looked over at Nigel; he was nonchalantly reading a newspaper. It seemed such a normal everyday task, on a day that felt far from routine. We locked up the house and headed back to the Care Home. I dreaded every second that we were approaching there. Upon our arrival back in the car park, we witnessed Judith's G.P. Dr. Allinson making his way to his car. He looked worried. Dealing with such cases as Judith's must be traumatic, even for a doctor, I thought. I wondered if he was shocked on seeing how Judith had mentally declined, so quickly. She had originally been with Dr. Allinson at the Ramsey Group Practice, but on moving to Laxey Glen

House Residential Home, she had also moved to a new G.P. in Laxey. When she moved back to Ramsey, Dr. Allinson had become her G.P. once again. He was a tall, pale, freckled man, with auburn-ginger hair and had a look of Boris Becker about him facially, from a distance. I guessed he was in his forties. He glanced at us in an almost apologetic, perhaps sympathetic, manner. Hours seemed to pass. Marie wandered out to see us once again. She had been back up to the third floor of the unit to sit with Judy and Jim. That time Judith had taken an instant dislike to Marie. Judith was convinced that Marie was having an affair with Jim, and, in Marie's words, Judith had called her, "A fucking slag", and had told her that she was not taking Jim away, and was not getting the house. Marie had no option but to retreat, as Judith became more aggressive and threatening in her nature. Marie asked us to return inside to the ground floor of the unit, as, while the doctors had both been visiting Judith and undertaking the Section 2, Marie had managed to get Jim away from Judy. We had all been most concerned for my father, over and above our concerns for Judith. I returned inside, just as my father exited the lift. The unit manager had accompanied him. They appeared hostile towards each other. My father looked completely drained. I attempted to hug him, but he pulled away. The strain had been all too much for him and tears rolled down his face. I moved in again and hugged him while he sobbed over my shoulder. He regained his composure, but with his chin quivering, and told me that he was now going home. I offered to accompany him back to his house, but he refused. He wanted to be alone, and he needed to rest. I doubted he would get any.

Marie promised that she would be in touch with my father later, to update him on Judith. My father hobbled out, leaning heavily on his walking stick; so frail and so ashen. I walked with him to his car and assisted him into the driver's seat. I was desperately sad for him. Such a proud man reduced to this.

We too needed to leave. The poor dog had been in the house all day. Although she had been walked before we left, she was now well overdue another walk, and her dinner too. The unit manager was still muttering about being there, "all night". I found myself disgusted with how long this Section and transfer had, and still was taking. Everybody concerned was exhausted, especially my father, who had been at high risk of another stroke. Nigel commented that they could not organise a piss-up in a brewery. The unit manager agreed. Normally I may have laughed, but humour was not abound. "Bloody ridiculous" was all I could manage.

At 9pm on 02 April 2012, Judith was eventually taken by ambulance to the unit. Her physical capacities at this point included eating and drinking for herself; fully mobile; toileting herself unaided when in the bathroom, and dressing herself with direction. Mentally, Judith was confused and agitated with high aggression. She recognised familiar faces at all times, and she remembered names too. She always carried a cuddly toy with her, and she was constantly talking to an imaginary person or children though.

10
Storm Damage

We arrived back home, both utterly depleted of energy. The mental strain was immense, and I could only sympathise about how my poor father was coping. Back from the nightmare that was, Kana jumped around yelping and barking when we entered the front door. Beaming her cute doggy smile and jumping up with such excitement. I immediately opened the back door and accompanied her into the garden. She squatted and relieved herself for a few long minutes, then promptly dashed around the garden like a crazed rabbit. So beautiful to see. In the midst of all the chaos of the day, she couldn't help but raise my spirits and a smile, from seeing her enthusiasm on our arrival back. Shani, the cat, had joined in too, leaping around and chasing her. Occasionally pouncing on her back and springing into the air. Later on, as I prepared dinner in the kitchen, the telephone rang. It was my father, who explained that Marie had called in on him to check that he was coping and to make sure that he had eaten. She informed him that Judy had calmed down at the unit now. She had eaten some dinner and was now sleeping. Marie advised that we should not visit Judy for a couple of days, to allow her time to settle down, without any external distractions. Judith was still expressing wishes to kill herself. My father told me that he may as well kill himself too. He was sick of dealing with everything and Judy was not his Judy anymore. He didn't want to live like this. He wished that he was dead.

I so wished that I could take his pain away. I tried my best to reason with him, telling him that a good night sleep would make everything a little brighter in the morning, and telling him that Judy needed us more than ever, to be strong for her. The professionals would help her, and she was in the right place for that. I asked him if he wanted to come and stay with us for a while, but he refused. He wanted to be alone, I told my father that I respected his decision, but the offer was always there. I had to stifle my tears on bidding him goodnight.

What a hideous surreal day it had been. Topped off with my father wishing to kill himself. My nerves were totally shot. I needed one huge glass of wine, or two, to take the edge off my anxiety. The tears were quietly rolling down my cheeks as I unscrewed the wine bottle. My appetite had vanished, but I continued to prepare the dinner, glugging down the wine in an attempt to anaesthetise the pressure of the day, and the sadness I felt for my parents. I would explain the situation to Sophie, my daughter, at the weekend. No need to bother her before then. Even as I drank my wine seeking some relief from the anxiety, my heart was heavy for my father. I was analysing the situation. Undoubtedly it had been the most horrendous day. For him to threaten suicide seemed to add salt to the raw open wounds, yet he had suffered a stroke that had left him physically weak, but had also changed him mentally too, with decreased sensitivity towards others and unquestionably weaker than the strong person that he once was. An untimely and disturbing predicament, to have both parents suffering almost parallel demises. As I quaffed my wine, one thing appeared certain; things were going to get a whole lot worse. I decided to numb the reality of the situation with a little more wine. Nigel could only reaffirm that I had once told him that I suspected that my mother had mental health issues for most of her life and that she would be a very difficult person if she ever developed dementia in later life. I understood that he was attempting to help me come to terms with the situation, but it felt more like, "Well, wham! There you go".

I decided to brave the cold and retreat to the garden. The temperature seemed preferable to the running commentary inside. Alone was when I was most comfortable with my own thoughts. Nigel had to let the dog out though. She wasn't going to allow me to have, "fun", in the garden, while she was stuck inside the house. I smiled as she scampered around the illuminated garden. Another click of the door, and out wandered the cat too. Animals had a wonderful way of knowing and comforting you in a time of upset. Such beautiful creatures – a true God send. I stood scrutinising the garden and looked up at the towering trees surrounding it. Everything was so perfectly made – the trees, the flowers, the grass, even the natural rocks in the rockery. Nothing was made by accident. They all had a perfect design; a purpose and a beauty. I was truly blessed to live in this outstanding world. In an unprecedented instance, I realised that we were given life for a reason. Good things given to make us appreciate, and bad things given as a challenge, with lessons to be learned from suffering difficulties. Bad made us cherish the good. Without bad there could be no comparison to good. We live and die. We laugh and cry. We love and hate. We nurture and kill. So much in the world that we do not understand. An ever-learning life, full of nature's complexities. We were given the human strengths to address them, and perhaps too many human weaknesses to ignore them. But we were ultimately given the freedom to decide on our choice of direction. The human mind can be our friend or our greatest enemy. As with any muscle, it needs training and guidance. Solitary deep thinking was so precious to me; a period of reflection and analysis. I felt re-energised by my own new sense of perspective.

The next few days were difficult. It was a case of ringing the unit and enquiring how Judith was. Each time it felt as if we were being given minimal routine updates. Judith had got up, showered, eaten breakfast, had juice and had slept well. She was constantly asking for Jim though. My father was supposed to abstain from visiting for two days, but he only managed the one day. He was desperate to see her and therefore on day two the unit allowed him to visit Judith. The Section 2 under the Mental Health Act 1998 in the Isle of Man meant that she was in legal custody of the Department of Health and that would be in place for two weeks. It was an emergency Section.

She was considered a risk to herself and a risk to others. Apparently, Judith was overjoyed to see Jim. She was kissing and cuddling him so much, that the nurses were concerned that she would topple him over with her enthusiasm, and they had to calm Judith down. She was then most anxious to determine if Jim had bought her any sweets. Thankfully he had. They sat in the lounge of the unit, and Judith offered the sweets around, to both staff and patients, before they headed off to Judy's room, where my father played some C.D's and assisted Judith to use the bathroom. My father remained for a couple of hours, but Judith was annoyed and fretful when he attempted to leave, causing quite a commotion. Staff had to use distraction techniques to facilitate Jim leaving.

My father later rang me to explain how distressing he found leaving Judy. He could hear her thumping on the security door and shouting, as he feebly walked to the exit of the unit. He hated leaving her, especially in that unit. Yet it was beyond his control. He told me that he wished he could just take her home. His voice quivered and broke, as he relayed this. Staff had to deal with the fall-out of Jim leaving on each occasion. Judith would be banging on the door, screaming and crying for Jim. I witnessed it numerous times and found it immensely disturbing. Yet when Jim arrived at the unit, it was ironically beautiful to see my mother race down the corridor to greet him, smothering him with gratitude and love. She never failed to tell him that she loved him. Jim would always reply that he loved her too. They were like two loved-up sweethearts. It was heartbreaking to watch. The adoration for each other was unrequited.

A few days later, I enquired with the unit if it was viable to bring Kana, the dog, to the car park in the unit and let Judith see her. It seemed almost cruel for her to be separated from the dog that she so loved. They were happy enough for this to happen, although I was a little apprehensive about seeing my mother again, hoping that she would have forgotten the animosity that she had towards me previously.

Thankfully, on entering the unit she ran to greet me, throwing her arms around me, saying, "Oh, Victoria", and embracing me. The first hurdle was uneventfully overcome.

I had explained to Judith that Kana had come to see her and was in the car. Judith became tearful and pleaded with me to take her to see the dog. We walked hand-in-hand out through the unit, to the car, being careful that she didn't trip, as she had on many occasions when she had stayed with me. (Once on the beach when walking Kana, Judith had tripped up, splaying on the floor and had then cried like a toddler, who had fallen over. Thankfully, there was no injury caused. Her walking was not hindered in the least bit, but sometimes her feet swelled, and this perhaps caused the slight shuffling that she had developed). Judith was ecstatic to see Kana, who was equally overjoyed to once again snuggle up to my mother. They both sat in the rear of the car getting reacquainted, before we all had a stroll around the car park. Surprisingly, when it came to the end of our visit, Judith was reasonably happy for Kana to return to the car, and for us to walk hand-in-hand back to the unit. No commotion and no refusal. The visit went even better than I had hoped for. I accompanied Judith to the residents' lounge where we both had a cup of tea. While Judith was preoccupied with watching television, I made my exit from the unit.

11

The Aftermath

My father visited my mother almost every day. I frequented, sometimes with Nigel, four or five times per week. Sophie, my daughter, visited at weekends, every other week.

Often, I would save magazines or specifically buy them, especially National Geographic magazine. We could then sit in the quiet room, with the relaxing bubble machine gently changing colour, and look at the pictures of animals and natural landscapes. Judith loved this, and we engaged in conversation regarding the images. Often my mother would stroke the pictures of the animals and become attached to these photographs. She always had her cuddly toy on her lap. It had become her comforter. Without it, she would become anxious. Perhaps it was her replacement for Kana, the Chihuahua. We nearly always had a cup of tea together, and Judith would love the biscuits accompanying it. She enjoyed her food and had a very healthy appetite. Jim would often bring her yoghurts or fresh fruit.

As the weeks passed by, Judith was very much up and down in her moods. Some days she would be relatively lucid when we visited, and at other times, very confused and frustrated. Both my father and I, when we visited, would ask Judith if she needed to use the bathroom. Both options were normally locked; the main toilet in the unit, and Judith's en-suite bathroom. We would have to ask a staff member for one to be unlocked if Judith did need to go. On one particular visit, I had taken my mother outside into the garden. As normal, we walked around admiring the flowers and birds. We then sat on a small bench together in the sunshine. After a couple of minutes Judith became anxious and tearful, and as I led her towards the main lounge, I could see that her trousers were saturated. I explained to one of the nurses that Judith had had an accident. She took my mother by the hand led her to her bedroom.

Sometime later, they both returned, with Judith in fresh trousers, and the nurse with a carrier bag containing the wet trousers, for me to launder. The nurse explained that Judith required some new trousers too, as she had ripped two pairs of trousers in anger, during the week. I agreed that I would bring in new trousers on my next visit.

I was a little disturbed to witness my mother's new acquired incontinence, but this incident was the start of many such occurrences. On one instance, when I visited Judith, I asked her if she wished to use the bathroom, which she indicated that she did. As I was leading her towards her room, Judith started pulling at her trousers frantically. I explained that she must wait until she was in her room, but she continued pulling at her waistband, angrily. I took this as a need for urgency, and quickened our pace, near dragging her by the hand. Once inside the room, I bent down and undid her button and zip on the trousers. To my surprise, she was wearing adult diapers. Yet, what shocked my more, was the fact that they had been fastened so very tightly. I had immense trouble trying to undo them. I assumed this would prove an almost impossible task for a dementia patient, as Judith too was distraughtly attempting to rip them off. Between us, we eventually ripped them off. It was impossible to unfasten them. I left my mother on the toilet, while I hurried off in search of her named nurse. I was angry at this point and questioned her as to why the diapers were so ridiculously tightly fastened. She retorted that Judith would take them off otherwise and her accidents were quite frequent. I stated that none of the available bathrooms should be locked either, but I was informed that it was due to patient safety, yet, I could see no valid reason for this. Seriously, what would patients do? Water-board themselves? Try to drown themselves in the toilet pan? Maybe I was missing something, but all patients had their belongings searched and sharp or hazardous items were removed. Even Judith's photo frames were not allowed in the unit, yet the toilets being locked made no sense at all, especially the main toilet in the unit.

On another occasion, I had helped my mother into her clean trousers, I had been shocked to witness the size of her calf muscles. They were so pronounced and reminded me of athletes, or footballers' legs. I could only relate this to her constant pacing of the corridors in the unit. I guessed she must be doing this for most of the day then. Quite a notable transformation I thought.

As Judith continued to be in the unit, her walking was becoming slower and she had a further pronounced shuffle, rather than her brisk, confident walk that she once had. She now moved like a cast-member from a zombie movie – a stiff-legged gait with small scraping steps and a definite hunched back. Where there was once a time during her earlier admittance to the unit, when she would run up the corridor, she would now hold onto the rail that ran parallel to the corridor wall. No expression on her face, and a vacant, dead-look in her eyes.

During one visit, Judith was moving around the main lounge with her cheek pressed against the wall, ensuring constant contact with it. As she attempted to manoeuvre around the corner of the room, she hit her nose flat against the adjacent wall, stumbling backwards in pain. Yet no words, or noise was made by Judith; her expression remained blank. It was heart wrenching to witness.

Staff were always present; maybe one, or sometimes two people, yet they appeared to be merely watchful of the patients, with little interaction. There appeared to be no activities, and little engagement with the patients. They were left to wander aimlessly. Bedroom doors and patients' bathrooms were normally locked, providing no free-access to toileting facilities. My school of thinking was that the toilet doors should have a large picture of a toilet displayed on it; easily recognisable for patients, especially those suffering with dementia.

Judith was in this unit, this second time, for just over three months. This followed her expulsion from the Laxey Glen House Residential

Home, and her subsequent first admittance to the unit. Although we were never advised of Judith's Care Plan, we were informed informally, by Marie, that, "they", were thinking of placing Judith in the Government run EMI (elderly mentally infirm), unit care home. My father was horrified on hearing this. He had visited this place with Judith and Marie, some months earlier, as a possible option. Judith had cried during the entire visit and begged my father not to leave her there. The experience of that unit had proved very traumatic for both of my parents. My mother was undoubtedly a very difficult case of a person with dementia. Although she was very robust physically at the time, her volatile mood-swings and aggression were exceptionally unpredictable. She was fully capable in body. She could walk and even run upon her second admission still; was able to feed herself, drink unaided and without prompting or direction. She was able to make a cup of tea for herself in the unit, with supervision, yet her constant companion was her cuddly toy whom she talked too, along with her imaginary friends. She was experiencing hallucinations too. Most disturbingly, Judith would become agitated when being assisted with the bathroom, or showering, often biting or scratching staff.

12

Devastating Losses

On 19 July 2012, some three and half months after her Section 2 admission to the unit, myself and my husband visited Judith in the unit as normal. On entering the unit, we were shown to where my mother was sitting, in a small seating area at the far end of the unit. When we reached her, it was immediately obvious that something was very wrong. She was sitting upright on the sofa, but she was leaning at an abnormal angle to the right-hand side, in an almost yoga-like side stretch. Her head was bent down with her chin nearly touching her chest. When I spoke to her, she never moved even an inch, but only groaned. I put my head underneath hers and looked into her eyes. She focused on me and her eyes widened in recognition. Her pupils were dilated. Again, she only made a pained murmur. She seemed unable to move and unable to speak.

I was alarmed and hurried off to find a member of staff. As I did so, I passed a Health Care Assistant, who, when I expressed my concern about Judith's condition, informed me that Judy's medication had been increased, to give her, "a well-earned rest". I enquired as to which medication had been increased, to which she replied that it was her diazepam, she thought. On asking a couple of the nursing staff about the increase in the medication, they could not confirm which drug, but assured me that it would have been Dr. Jagus, her Psychiatrist who would have increased any of her medication, as he saw fit, as Judith had become even more distressed. Nobody appeared to see the unusual posture that was concerning me the most.

I returned to sit with my mother, still concerned by her condition.

The afternoon tea trolley came around and the apologetic-looking lady gave Judith her usual cup of tea, placing it on the table in front of her. At this point, I explained to the lady, that my mother was in no fit state to drink unaided, and I expressed my concern about her becoming dehydrated. When the tea had cooled, I attempted to encourage Judith to take a sip by placing the cup to her sideways mouth, although it was clear from the angle of her head, that she would be unable to drink. Her eyes were straining to make contact with mine. She was struggling to speak, but she managed only low moans or "ah". Did I see an expression of needing help in her eyes, or was she just so drugged up? I was so shocked and immensely worried by what I witnessed. Judith was in dire need of medical intervention. Various staff members from the unit came to reassure me that Judith was sedated and needed the "time-out", from her distress. I could neither argue the case or expand further on my concern and anxiety that I was experiencing over her posture and physical state. On leaving the unit, I voiced my concern to a male nurse, about my mother becoming dehydrated. He in turn, assured me that they would give her water. My husband attempted to dispel my fears, by assuring me that the unit dealt with these situations every day.

We travelled home in almost silence. The long, winding country lanes seemed to continue forever. Even the beauty of the greenery could not lift my spirits. I was deeply worried and perplexed by my mother's condition.

I barely slept that night. When I had eventually fallen asleep, I had awoken in a state of panic and tearfulness. Nigel's patience was running thin; evidenced in his tone with me. I explained that there was something desperately wrong with my mother's condition. In the heat-of-the-moment, he called my mother, "mental", and asked me if I was a doctor. I despised him for ridiculing both myself and my mother. I remember just screaming at him to, "fuck off". He attempted to back-peddle and cuddle me. I pushed him away and spat, "Do not touch me". I tried to feign sleep, and turned my back to him. It felt as if he had just stuck a knife into me when I was almost on the floor already.

The sunlight spilled into the bedroom at dawn. The birds were already cheerfully singing. I wanted to stay in bed; never wake up. Anxiety and a sense of fear had a firm grip on me. I struggled, depleted of energy, to take a shower, but felt somewhat better after taking one. It was maybe nearly midday when my father telephoned. Judith was being transferred to the medical ward at Noble's hospital. He sounded flat in his manner, and very "matter-of-fact"; at his wits end. He was presently at the unit with my mother and explained that she was in bed unable to move or speak to him. I reassured him that I would go to the unit immediately.

I went out to the garden and into the outbuildings to find Nigel. I explained the situation to him. He in return insisted on going with me too. I informed him that his presence with me was neither helpful, nor necessary. He offered no opposition. He understood that my, "fuck off" still stood.

The drive to the unit, seemed to take so long. My heart was racing; my throat tighter than ever and my legs were having problems with the car pedals – my legs had turned to quivering jelly. I had a sense of pure fear surrounding me.

On entering my mother's unit, two nurses – one male, one female, rushed towards me in a panic and ushered me towards my mother's bedroom. I met my bewildered father in the corridor. He was deathly pale with a grey tone to his face. I hugged him and he explained that he needed to return home, now that I had arrived. I tried to dispel his worries and kissed him goodbye. I would call him later to update him on Judy. He really needed to rest up as he looked so ill. The male nurse accompanied my father out. The female, Nurse Halsall led me inside the bedroom of my mother. My instant reaction was, "What the hell?".

Judith's head was twisted sideways, nearly touching her right shoulder. Most noticeable was the swelling to her neck, face and forearms. Her skin looked so pale and white, resembling that of a deceased person. She was unable to talk, only mumble, as if her mouth was full of tissue. She could not move at all. The only parts of her body that she moved were her eyes in her fixed head, and her hands, but only from her wrists. Her lips were visibly crusted and her tongue, which occasionally poked out from her mouth, was dry and cracked also. Her forearms appeared body-builder-like, as I had previously witnessed in the calf of her legs on 30 May 2012. By now I was in no mood for pleasantries. I sternly told Nurse Halsall that my mother was dehydrated and required water to drink. She went to fetch water and returned with water in a beaker with a spout. I attempted to give Judith water, but as I cupped the back of her neck to raise it to the beaker, she shrieked in agony. Why such pain in the neck?

The nurse elevated the headrest on the bed. Judith started shrieking again, with a near audible muffled cry of, "No". The nurse quickly reclined the bed again. Nurse Halsall explained that they had tried to give Judith a drink, but that she had refused it. This alarmed me, as quite clearly my mother was totally "unable", to drink. She further explained that Judith had developed a rash on both legs, and that was the reason for the awaited transfer to Noble's Hospital. I reiterated that I was more concerned by the swelling in her neck and around her face. Judith's skin looked so tightly stretched over her cheekbones. Her eyes were wide-open like a scared rabbit. Nurse Halsall explained that the ambulance might be some time, and then left the room.

I removed the spout from the beaker and attempted to pour some water into Judith's mouth, being careful not to choke her. She closed her eyes for a couple of seconds, in what appeared to be relief. As I pulled the cup away from her mouth, she managed to grip my hand on the way down. She dug her nails into my hand. I looked at her face. She was trying to talk, but she managed only groans. Her eyes looked pleading with me. "What the hell was going on?", I thought.

The nurse re-entered the room and informed me that I was likely to choke Judith by pouring water into her mouth. She explained to me that they used to be able to re-hydrate patients by soaking sterile gauze with water, then wringing it into the patient's mouth, but this was no longer policy. I felt slightly irritated by this. I didn't want to hear about what they, "used to do". I was only interested in the moment.......now.

I searched through Judith's bedroom locker and found two white, unused flannels. I soaked them both in cold water and placed one on my mother's forehead, as she was sweating, then rung the other into her mouth. Again, a flicker of relief in Judith's eyes. I repeated this process for well over an hour. As I slowly attempted to rehydrate my mother, her mumbling became louder and more agitated. She was becoming more alert, yet there was still no further movement in her body. I was very, very, concerned.

Nurse Halsall returned again and told me that the ambulance may still be some time, due to the fact that Judith was effectively already in a hospital environment, and she required a "transfer" only. I again expressed my worries over the swelling, and she retorted, "Something is certainly not being addressed". She advised me that she would be accompanying my mother to the hospital and that I should leave and visit her there later. I agreed with this and told Nurse Halsall that once the formal admission of Judith into Noble's Hospital had been completed and she was settled, then I would visit my mother later that evening.

I drove back to my house totally bewildered and anxious about the whole situation. I questioned myself, as to whether I was being overly dramatic and concerned, as there seemed to be no sense of urgency from the staff at the unit. Judith had lost her speech, total mobility, her ability to eat or drink and her physical condition with the increased muscle bulk, was appalling. All of which had happened over a period of twenty-four hours or so. When I reached my house, I immediately telephoned my father to update him on Judy's predicament. My father was convinced that my mother was suffering from mumps or glandular fever. I said that I thought that there might be a drug interaction, or something similar, but again impressed that Judy was in the right place to get diagnosed, as they would run tests to determine the cause. This was the first time that he criticised the unit staff, saying all they seemed to do was sit around watching television, or sorting paperwork. He was fretful and understandably angry.

Judith was to be moved to Ward 2 – the female admissions ward. Upon telephoning them, through the main hospital switchboard, after a little confusion, I was advised that she had been admitted to Ward 1 – the male admissions ward, as Ward 2 was fully occupied. It was nearing 7pm when I was advised that Judith was, "settled in".

I made my way to the ward as quickly as possible. On arrival, the nursing staff showed me to my mother's bed. She appeared to be no different than she had been at the unit. Still with her head lolling to one-side in a most uncomfortable nature. She was sleeping – or near unconscious – it was difficult to tell. Occasionally, her legs went into a seizure-type shaking, but only for a matter of seconds. Most disturbingly, she was not on I.V. fluids. I asked the nurse present why this was. She assured me that this would be completed later, after the doctor had seen her. Again, I was disturbed. My mother had been waiting to be admitted to the hospital since at least 10 a.m. that day, having received no fluid, apart from the water I had earlier given to her. There seemed to be no sense of urgency, despite the fact that Judith had lost all mobility; could not talk and now appeared barely conscious, with swelling around her neck, face and forearms; not to mention the hideous contortion of the neck – all of which I raised concerns about with the nurse present that evening. Sadly, there appeared to be little point in me staying for any great length of time, as my mother was not rousable.

I decided to make my way home, yet really not wanting to leave due to my apprehension about her condition.

It was approaching dark outside and very windy. When I arrived home the trees were swaying and creaking in the garden. The dog Kana was overjoyed to see me, which again lifted my mood somewhat.

After making a big fuss of her, I telephone my father to further update him on Judith's situation. He had convinced himself that Judy had mumps. I expressed my scepticism on this.

We arranged to meet during visiting hours the following day. I could hear by the tone of his voice, that he was exhausted.

13

The Loss Adjusters

My father and I visited Judith in the medical ward every day. Jim travelled once a day, and due to the proximity of the hospital to my house, I visited twice a day. The journey via the country lanes, took between ten and fifteen minutes by car.

For days Judith was so drowsy that neither of us witnessed her awake. He head was still at the unusual side-angle. Each time I visited her the pillow was central to her bed, yet her head was to one-side. I adjusted her pillow each visit to support her head.

During her time on this ward, the eventual and presumed diagnosis was pyelonephritis – kidney infection. No urinalysis was performed though. An enlarged kidney was noted on an ultrascan, but was otherwise noted as, "unremarkable". An abnormal E.C.G was noted.

Judith was pyrexia, (high temperature), prior to her admission. She had very little urine output noted too. Her liver function tests showed raised levels of Gamma Glutamyl Transferase. This was also raised in her bone profile.

Electrolyte tests revealed high levels of C Reactive Protein; an indicator of liver inflammation. Liver function tests revealed high levels of albumin, the day after her hospital admission. All levels continued to rise further. Yet still no urinalysis was performed.

Prior to this admission, Judith had been identified as having a urinary tract infection; E-choli resistant, on 12 July 2012. She was known to have previous hepatic impairment.

Upon admission her prescribed medication was:-

Diazepam	5mg	TDS
Procyclidine	2.5mg	TDS
Lactulose	10ml	BD
Lanzoprazole	80mg	OD
Donezepil	10mg	OD
Furosemide	20mg	OD
Pregablin	25mg	BD
Risperidone	0.5mg	BD
Sodium Valproate	100mg	TDS
Mirtazapine	45mg	ON

A review of her medication was requested by the ward, but no alteration was made to Judith's prescription. Also noted in Judith's medical records, by a Psychiatrist, Dr Slater, was that Judith was in, "danger of polypharmacy". Meaning in danger of "concurrent use of multiple medications by a patient". "Danger – "likely to cause harm or injury" or at the very least, danger means, "the possibility of something unwelcome, harmful or unpleasant happening".

On day three of Judith's admission, I visited my mother and was met by the Ward Sister, who informed me that Judith was ready to be discharged back to Grianagh Court, the mental health unit, but the Sister was disgusted that the unit didn't have a bed free for Judith. I argued that my mother could not possibly be ready for discharge. She was in a near-coma; couldn't walk, talk, or even eat and drink. All of which were capabilities lost within a matter of twenty-four hours or so. She then went on to inform me that they were unaware of any of these issues and they were only dealing with an infection. I stated that I was now making her aware of these issues and that my mother should not be discharged. Regardless of this, Judith was discharged back to the Mental Health Unit on 27 July 2012, in the evening, when a bed became free again. It was very clear to our family that she was not fit for discharge. Her condition remained unchanged from the first day of her admission to the medical ward.

The next time I saw my mother after her discharge back to the EMI unit, was the following morning.

That very next morning I arrived at the unit expecting a marked improvement in my mother; albeit a miracle would have happened. Yet I was even more shocked when I actually saw her. She was lying in bed. Still unrousable and with the swelling in her face, neck and forearms. There was no change at all. Judith was unable to move; talk, eat; drink. Her single bed had no bed rails. One side of the bed was pushed against the magnolia coloured wall. The open side of the bed had a rubber mat slung on the floor below it; obviously to cushion her fall if she did fall out. I was appalled at her condition. She clearly could not drink and was without means of rehydration, yet again. I was at boiling point. I am aware that I am on the "spectrum", so had to take serious stock of myself, yet I was trembling with anger. I told the male nurse present that, "A blind man with a stick and dog can see that she is seriously ill". Thankfully he agreed with me. He went off and returned with my mother's named nurse, Delia, whom myself, my husband and my father had met one week previously to request a meeting with my mother's psychiatrist, Dr. Jagus, which incidentally never happened, despite repeated requests.

I insisted that my mother was gravely ill and needed to see a doctor immediately. I expressed my opinion that Judith was suffering from an adverse drug reaction. (it is important to emphasise that I, and indeed my father, had no idea of the medication that was currently being prescribed to my mother, apart from the diazepam Judith required sometimes to calm her down). No discussions about medication had taken place on either occasion whilst Judith was in the unit. No adverse effects had been mentioned and certainly, no increase of mortality associated with the any medication was addressed. The nurse, Delia, explained that a doctor was making his rounds and would see my mother shortly.

Perhaps some half-an-hour later, a man came into my mother's bedroom, followed by Delia. I was shocked when I turned to see who had entered the room. This man was dressed in full black, waterproof motorcycle attire, except for the crash helmet. He looked threatening dressed like this to me, let alone to a mentally ill patient. To me it was inappropriate to visit this unit as he was. In my mind I was thinking, "You totally disrespectful, insensitive idiot". Beyond my belief and comprehension. I saw my mother's eyes widen as he approached her. She started to moan and attempted to shout. I took her hand to reassure her. I touched around her throat and neck, explaining to this doctor that these areas were unusually swollen. I explained that she had become totally bed-bound and was unable to speak, just recently, only the last week, and this total incapacitation had happened over a period of maybe less than twenty-four hours. I had no expectations of his response, but I was aghast when he flatly remarked that he was just a," community doctor", and that there was nothing he could do. I looked him in the eyes, smiled sweetly and said, "It is clear to me that you are a very busy man and need to be elsewhere, instead of here".

I turned, walked out of the door and stood outside raging with frustration. What exactly was he here to do?

He came out of my mother's bedroom, acknowledged me, and left. I re-entered Judith's room and informed Delia that I still wanted the meeting with Judith's Psychiatrist, Dr. Jagus. Delia had rung me at my home, one week earlier to ask if I still wanted to have a meeting with him. I had confirmed that I did, yet nothing was arranged. I relayed to Delia bluntly, that I was not happy with my mother's condition and felt that they were all failing her. She needed to be in a medical ward. She rushed out, then returned after a few minutes to inform me that another doctor would be visiting Judith later on.

At this point I decided to return home. I was aware that I was feeling distressed, angry and frustrated. I was in dire need of removing myself from the present situation. I was on the verge of, "losing it". My whole body was shaking with pure anger. A male nurse confronted me on the way out and explained that they were unhappy with Judith's condition too. I merely shook my head in dismay, and I left. I would return later when I had calmed down. I was stunned by their attitude in the unit; shocked beyond belief, but most of all angry and frustrated by them.

On arrival home, despite the drive back, I was still fuming. Relaying her condition and the events at the unit to Nigel didn't ease the frustration. He assured me that they would have performed all the necessary tests on her and asked me if I knew more than the doctors. He heightened my anxiety. I found myself screaming that something was wrong with my mother, telling him that, "Mr Fucking Nice Guy", just accepted things – never wanted to question or cause a commotion – had no backbone- was useless and unsupportive". I had to catch myself. I was at exploding point; wanted to throw things; trash stuff. My whole body was shaking and my knees were weak. My heart was pounding and I could feel the veins bulging under pressure in my neck, with the sheer tension I was experiencing. I ran upstairs and locked myself in a bedroom and shouted, "Fuck off", every time Nigel banged on the door. I was in melt-down. Jesus, this was all I needed – me out of control. I lay down on the bed, sobbing like a distraught toddler, curled up in a foetal position, hugging my knees.

I was awoken sometime later by a knock on the door. I had calmed down. The, "fuck off", was replaced with a sullen, "What?". Nigel explained that my father was on the telephone. I jumped up quickly, opened the door and took the phone from Nigel. My father explained that they were moving Judy back to Noble's Hospital medical ward again. That was on 27 July 2012.

This time I wanted to be with my mother as soon as she was being admitted. I asked the unit which ward she would be admitted too. I then telephoned that ward and asked them to telephone me, when Judith arrived for formal admission.

When the ward called me upon her arrival, I headed to the hospital by myself in the car. A mix of emotions was flooding through me. Panic; distress; anxiety, frustration, but most prevalent was anger. Nobody at the Mental Health Unit seemed to have a clue about Patient Safety, and more worryingly, they didn't seem to care. All the time there was an air of arrogance about most of the staff – as if they were doing everybody a favour. I could almost see the huge chip on their shoulders. I had spoken to a few staff members, and it was clear that they were disgruntled by their lack of pay. Perhaps they were underpaid for their roles – less than the UK, they led me to believe, but they were paid and had willingly engaged in accepting their professional positions and responsibilities associated with them.

Again, a panic-type attack set in. Tight chest; tight bulging throat feeling; sweating palms; racing heartbeat and trembling legs. I knew that my blood pressure was sky high of late. My G.P. had given me beta-blockers in an attempt to reduce it. The once situational high blood pressure, stress and anxiety were now a daily occurrence. I could only imagine how my poor father was coping.

Once again, I eventually parked the car in the over-full car park and headed towards the main hospital doors. I asked at reception for the directions to the admission ward, and followed the directions given. I found Judith being attended by a rather young-looking and nervous doctor in a hijab. My mother was in a highly anxious state. No different to exactly one week previously. Still the swelling in her neck, face and forearms. Still with her head twisted sideways and unable to move or talk – just groans and muffled noises, occasionally poking her tongue out, in a grimace. The only body parts she could move were her hands, but only from the wrists still, along with her eyes and her mouth, just slightly. Strangely, my mother was shrieking every time she merely anticipated the doctor touching or contacting with her hands, as if they were painful.

Every time my mother could grasp the doctor's hand, Judith would attempt to dig her nails into them. I had to keep releasing her grip, to allow the doctor to perform her duties. I explained to the doctor about the unusual swelling in Judith's face and neck, and told her about the recently acquired state of Judith, being unable to move, eat or talk. The doctor seemed neither surprised, nor in fact, interested. She made a phone call during which she commented that the patient was hitting her. I was thinking of contradicting her and explaining that Judith was in a state of panic, was not actually hitting her, as she was not capable of that in her current state, but I saw the exercise as pointless. The doctor then turned to me and explained that they would need to perform urinalysis on my mother, and then proceeded to ask me how she should get the urine. I think at this point, I was stunned and may have even laughed. But I do remember saying, "You are the doctor. You must have done this before". In truth my heart just sank. Jesus, who was extracting the urine indeed?

During the first visiting hours the next day, I visited my mother. There was no improvement in her condition. She was on the I.V. fluids, but her food intake was minimal, mainly due to drowsiness and being asleep for the majority of the day.

I spoke with the nurses on the desk again and asked about Judith's diagnosis. They informed me that it was probably cholecystitis – inflammation of the gallbladder; in this case due to gall stones, which was a condition that had been identified some months, if not a year ago, in Judith, yet no treatment had been deemed necessary. My mother was to be prescribed further antibiotics. For a period in excess of two weeks Judith had been undergoing treatment with various antibiotics. I found myself bewildered as to why a simple diagnosis of gall stones had taken so long. Yet it didn't seem plausible to me that it would cause my mother to lose all capacity and be rendered into a vegetative state, with the swelling in her neck, face and forearms, or the twisted angle of her neck. Nothing was making sense to me.

Later that evening when I visited my mother in the ward, I was alarmed to see that her bed was empty and had been freshly made. My heart skipped a beat. A nurse had recognised me and came walking over. She must have seen the flicker of shock on my face. She informed me that they had moved Judith from the Medical Assessment Ward to Ward 5. This was on 29 July 2012.

14
Uninsured

I would visit my mother twice a day, and my poor father would visit once a day, but he stayed for a couple of hours at least. Judith was catheterised and was on I.V. fluids. Her food intake was self-limited to a mouthful or two of food each day. She was particularly drowsy and slept most of the day and night still. We saw no improvement in her presentation.

I was becoming more and more concerned as the days passed, and would ask everyday why there was no improvement in Judith's condition. They had no idea and were still doing ongoing investigations. Nobody in the hospital could provide any answers as to why Judith's balance had gone too. The doctor had attempted to sit her up in a chair, but she would only fall sideways like a new baby. She appeared to be in pain and was unable to adopt a straight posture at all. She struggled with staying awake. She was constantly sleeping.

On another occasion, two staff nurses came over to me for a "quick word". They explained that sometimes the dementia drugs that were given to dementia patients could, in all honesty, cause more harm than good. Some were in fact dangerous. I was quite taken aback. I asked the staff nurses which drugs in particular they were referring to. They told me the name, then I requested them to write it down for me. They wrote the word RISPERIDONE.

Over the past week or so, I had been trying to search the internet for any lead that might offer an insight in my mother's condition. Mostly, I had typed swelling of the neck and face, but it was too random to find any result. It was simply like finding a needle in a haystack, so to speak. It had become my all consuming passion, and Nigel had become infuriated with me, asking if I was studying to become a doctor. Yet I was totally convinced that there was something crucial being missed with my mother. Judith was becoming weaker by the day and refusing all but a mouthful or two of food. It was as if she suddenly remembered that she was on a diet, then point-blank refusing to eat anything further.

I raced home with new hope, eager to do more digging, armed with this new information. As soon as I arrived home, I relayed to Nigel the conversation that I had with the two staff nurses during the visit. I opened my laptop, at which point Nigel began with his tirade, ranting about spending all my time on the internet, thinking I knew more than the doctors, complaining that we were not spending any quality time together. The verbal onslaught was too much. I was screaming, "What the fuck is up with you? You have seen my mother's condition – there is something very wrong with her". His bitterness was overwhelming. I picked up my laptop, stormed upstairs and locked the bedroom door. I would not be bullied into submission. I researched Risperidone – an antipsychotic medication. Words like, "danger", "caution", "Black-box warning", jumped out at me. Serious side-effects in dementia patients became evident. Alarm bells were ringing loudly already. I scrolled on the internet for hours, noting the hazardous warnings about this Risperidone in the use of the elderly and especially in elderly dementia patients. After reading many articles, my next move was to find a Patient Information Leaflet on Risperidone. That was on my agenda as a priority, for the next day. I would head to my local pharmacy and ask if they could provide me with one. This would be essential to my further understanding of the implications of this medication.

The following morning I visited the said chemist and asked if it was possible to obtain a Patient Information Leaflet for Risperidone. They informed me that they could not allow me to take one, as the P.I.L. had to accompany the medicine on prescription, but the Pharmacist was helpful enough to explain that I could download one from the internet. I was due to visit my mother in a couple of hours, so I would obtain the leaflet by download later, after visiting Judith in the evening. Yet I was anxious to know what was wrong with my mother and the implications, if any, for her future health.

Every day, I would ask the nursing staff for an update, if any, on Judith's condition. They were quite honest with me – they didn't know what was causing her drowsiness, loss of balance and loss of mobility. They seemed as frustrated as I was. One Consultant advised that he wished for my mother's Consultant Psychiatrist to visit her for a further assessment. He apparently visited her on 31 July 2012. Unbeknown to us at the time, Dr Jagus then discontinued Judith's prescribed Pregablin and Risperidone. The Diazepam was to be reduced from 5mg three times a day, to 2mg This was due to concerns about her drowsiness. She was to continue with her prescription of Sodium Valproate 100mg three times a day. For the next week, Judith was on I.V fluids and concern was raised about her nutritional intake.

My Risperidone research commenced with the download from the internet of the Patient Information Leaflet, as the pharmacist had recommended. Risperidone was under the brand name Risperdal. I learned that it is an antipsychotic drug, used in the treatment of schizophrenia, mania and for the short-term use (up to six weeks), of long-term aggression in people with Alzheimer's dementia, who harm themselves or others. Alternative, (non-drug), treatments should have been used previously. It was also used for short-term treatment, (up to six weeks), of long-term aggression in intellectually disabled children, 5 years and over, and adolescents with conduct disorder.

This is not an exhaustive context of the Patient Information Leaflet:-

When taking Risperidone, special care must be taken if:-

You have a heart problem.

You are at risk of a stroke.

You have ever experienced involuntary movement of the tongue, mouth and face.

You have ever had a condition whose symptoms include high temperature, muscle stiffness, sweating or a lowered level of consciousness (also known as Neuroleptic Malignant Syndrome).

You have Parkinson's disease or dementia.

You have kidney problems.

You have liver problems.

It is especially important to talk to your doctor or pharmacist if you are taking any of the following:-

Medicines that work on your brain such as to help you calm down (benzodiazepines), or some medicines for pain, (opiates), medicines for allergy, (some antihistamines), some antidepressants or other medicine for mental problems.

Medicines that cause a slow heartbeat.

Medicines that cause low blood potassium, (certain diuretics).

Medicines to treat raised blood pressure. Risperdal can lower blood pressure.

Medicines for Parkinson's disease.

Water tablets (diuretics), used for heart problems or swelling of parts of your body due to a buildup of too much fluid, (such as furosemide or chlorothiazide). Risperdal taken by itself or with furosemide may have an increased risk of stroke or death in elderly people with dementia.

People with liver or kidney problems.

Regardless of the disease to be treated, all starting doses and following doses of Risperidone should be halved.

Dose increase should be slower in these patients.

Risperidone should be used with caution in this patient group.

Possible Side Effects:-

Like all medicines, Risperdal can cause side effects, although not everybody gets them.

Tell your doctor immediately if you:-

Experience blood clots in the veins, especially in the leg.

Have dementia and experience a sudden change in your mental state, or sudden weakness or numbness of your face, arms or legs, especially on one side, or slurred speech, even for a short period of time. These may be signs of a stroke.

Experience fever, muscle stiffness, sweating or lowered level of consciousness, (a disorder called Neuroleptic Malignant Syndrome). Immediate medical treatment may be needed.

Experience involuntary movement of the tongue, mouth and face. Withdrawal of risperidone may be needed.

The following side effects may happen:-

Very common, (affects more than 1 in 10).

Parkinsonism. This is a medical term that includes many symptoms. Each individual symptom may occur less frequently than 1 in 10 people.

Parkinsonism includes: increase in saliva secretion or watery, musculoskeletal stiffness, drooling, jerks when bending limbs, slow, reduced or impaired body movements, no expression on the face, muscle tightness, stiff neck, muscle stiffness; small, shuffling, hurried steps and lack of normal arm movement when walking; persistent blinking in response to tapping of the forehead, (an abnormal reflex).

Headache, difficulty falling or staying asleep.

Common, (affects 1 in 10 users in 100).

Drowsiness, fatigue, restlessness, inability to sit still, irritability, anxiety, sleepiness, dizziness, poor attention, feeling exhausted, sleep disorder.

Vomiting, diarrhoea, constipation, nausea, increased appetite, decreased appetite, abdominal pain or discomfort, sore throat, dry mouth.

Difficulty breathing, lung infection, (pneumonia), flu, infection of the breathing passage, blurred vision, nose congestion, nose bleeding, cough.

Urinary tract infection, bed wetting.

Tremor, muscle spasm, involuntary movement of face or arms and legs.

Rash, skin redness.

Fast beating heart, chest pain.

Blood prolactin hormone level increase.

Uncommon, (affects 1 in 10 users in 1,000).

Excessive drinking of water, stool incontinence, thirsty, very hard faeces, hoarseness or voice disorder.

Diabetes, mellitus, high blood sugar.

Lung infection caused by inhaling food into the breathing passages, bladder infection, “pink eye”, sinus infection, eye discharge, yeast infection of the nails.

Abnormal electrical conduction of the heart, drop in blood pressure after standing, low blood pressure, feeling dizzy after changing body position, abnormal electric activity tracing of the heart, (ECG), abnormal heart rhythm, awareness of heart beating, heart rate increased or decreased.

Urinary incontinence, pain when passing urine, frequent passing of urine.

Confused, disturbance in attention, low level of consciousness, excessive sleep, nervousness, elated mood, (mania), lack of energy and interest.

Liver enzyme increased, white blood cell count decreased, (including those that help to protect you against bacterial infections), low haemoglobin or red blood cell count, (anaemia), increase in eosinophils, (special white blood cells), blood creatine phosphokinase increased, decrease in platelets, (blood cells that help you stop bleeding), increased blood cholesterol and triglycerides, (blood fats).

Muscle weakness, muscle pain, ear pain, neck pain, joint swelling, abnormal posture, joint stiffness, musculoskeletal chest pain, chest discomfort.

Skin lesion, skin disorder, dry skin, intense itching of the skin, acne, hair loss, skin inflammation caused by mites, skin discolouration, thickening of skin, flushing, reduced skin sensitivity to pain or touch, inflammation of oily skin.

No menstruation, sexual dysfunction, ejaculation disorder, breast discharge, enlargement of breasts in men, decreased sexual drive, irregular menstruation, vaginal discharge.

Fainting, gait disturbance, sluggishness, decreased appetite resulting in malnutrition and low body weight, feeling "out of sorts", balance disorder, allergy, oedema, speech disorder, chills, abnormal coordination, abnormal taste.

Painful oversensitivity to light, increased blood flow to the eye, eye swelling, dry eye, increase in tears.

Breathing passage disorder, lung congestion, crackly lung noise, congestion of breathing passages, trouble speaking.

Rare (affection 1 to 10 in 10,000).

Infection.

Inappropriate secretion of hormone that controls urine volume.

Sugar in urine, Low blood sugar.

Neuroleptic Malignant Syndrome, confusion, reduced or loss of consciousness, high fever and severe muscle stiffness.

Blood vessel problems in the brain.

Breakdown of muscle fibres and pain in muscles, (rhabdomyolysis).

Tremor of the head.

Coma due to uncontrolled diabetes.

My head was reeling from the intake of information. I had no idea that prescribed medication could have so many dangerous, potential side effects. Why would a doctor prescribe this medication to elderly dementia patients, who might already have communication issues due to dementia?

On reading the literature, two things were immediately apparent. Firstly, the heightened dangers of risperidone in elderly dementia patients was clearly potentially dangerous and secondly, none of these possible reactions detailed, could explain my mother's presentation at present.

I re-read the information many times. All of the detailed side-effects I understood, except for the one called, "Neuroleptic Malignant Syndrome". I had never heard of this.

15
Bearing the Costs

For many days during our visits to Judith there was little change in her condition. Her food and liquid intake were negligible, and her weight was dropping continuously. She was refusing to eat, and on occasions she would physically spit the second mouthful of food out.

A differential diagnosis of encephalitis or multiple strokes was made, but following a C.T. scan, M.R.I. scan and a lumbar puncture, this was discounted. The doctors informed us that they had no explanation for Judith's drowsiness, immobility and lack of balance. A doctor noted my mother as showing signs of Babinksi reflex – this is an important neurological examination based upon what the big toe does. If the big toe goes up it is a sign of a problem. Most newborn babies are not neurologically mature, so they normally have a Babinski sign, but a Babinski sign in an older child or adult is abnormal. It is a signal that a problem is in the central nervous system (CNS), most likely in the part called the pyramidal tract. (Ref: Medical Definition of Babinski Sign. Medical Author: William C. Shiel Jr., MD, FACP, FACR).

On 07 August 2012, Judith was given a Nasal Gastric tube to allow feeding to be administered, and she remained on I.V. fluids. I met with one of her Consultants, Dr. Majeed and asked him if it was possible that my mother had suffered from Neuroleptic Malignant Syndrome, as a result of her prescribed risperidone. He informed me that this was a possibility. Although I remained outwardly calm in his presence, I was astounded to hear this. He further confirmed, again, that they could find no explanation for Judith's condition, but that her risperidone had been stopped and her condition should improve.

The main difficulty with the N.G. tube for feeding, was that although my mother was still immobile and mute, she had gained a little more movement in her arms, since the swelling in her face, neck and arms had depleted over those last few days. Sadly, due to her confused state still, she kept dislodging the N.G. tube. Replacing it each time was distressing her too.

On 13 August 2012, we later found out, that her prescribed medication of Diazepam Mirtazapine and Donepezil was stopped, as Judith was opening her eyes in response to pain stimuli only. The Psychiatrist thought it was possible that these drugs were causing her drowsiness.

By 14 August 2012, Judith was rousable, responding to vocal commands by opening her eyes.

On 20 August 2012, the ward referred Judith back to Grianagh Court for further care, as she was much more alert, feeling better and more responsive. Medically, there was nothing more the ward could do for Judith. She was still drowsy and immobile. Her Consultant Psychiatrist, Dr. Jagus advised of a gradual reduction of her Sodium Valproate by 100mg each dose time.

Judith had now been bed-bound for one month.

My mother's Care Worker, Marie, came into the ward and explained to us that Judith was due to be discharged back to the EMI unit, at Grianagh Court; my father was present too. Firstly, my father and I were shocked to hear this. It was, without a doubt, clear to us that Judith was still exceptionally poorly. She had an N.G. tube in place and was on I.V fluid, with no mobility or balance. I demanded a meeting with her Psychiatrist, Dr Jagus. I told Marie, in no uncertain terms, that what the unit had done to my mother was diabolical, and I held them personally responsible for Judith's condition.

I was fed-up with pussy footing around. I had more insight into Judith's condition now, and I understood the increased high chance of her mortality associated with it. In that split second, I was determined to take the matter further and start with a letter of complaint to the Mental Health Services. My poor father was just welling up with tears. I wanted to protect him as much as possible from any stress, but there was no way that he would allow Judith to return to that unit.

Further to my research on Neuroleptic Malignant Syndrome, various articles came to my attention. Interestingly, the United States has an emergency twenty four hour hotline for questions, or for sufferers of the condition, called The Neuroleptic Malignant Syndrome Information Service who say, "The recognition, diagnosis and treatment of NMS and related hyperthermic disorders, is critical in avoiding morbidity and mortality. (www.mhaus.org/nmsis)

My research disclosed that:-

Neuroleptic Malignant Syndrome (NMS), is a life-threatening neurologic emergency associated with the use of neuroleptic agents.

Mortality results directly from dysautonomic manifestations of the disease and systemic complications. Mortality has declined from the earliest reports of the 1960's of 76 percent and is more recently estimated at 10-20 percent. This probably reflects greater awareness of the disease, earlier diagnosis and more aggressive intervention.

Both "typical" antipsychotic agents and the newer "atypical," antipsychotic drugs, (of which risperidone is), have been implicated in NMS.

While symptoms normally develop during the first two weeks of narcoleptic therapy, the association of the syndrome with the drug is idiosyncratic.

Typical symptoms – the tetrad of NMS symptoms typically evolve over a one to three day period.

Mental status change is the initial symptom in 82% of patients. This often takes the form of an agitated delirium with confusion rather than psychosis. Catatonic signs and mutism can be prominent. Evolution to profound encephalopathy with stupor and coma is typical.

Muscular rigidity is generalised and is often extreme. The increased tone can be demonstrated by moving extremities and is characterised by, "lead pipe rigidity" or stable resistance through all ranges of movement. Superimposed tremor may lead to a racketing quality, or a cogwheel phenomenon.

Other motor abnormalities include tremor (seen in 45 to 92 %) and less commonly dystonia, (involuntary muscle contractions that cause repetitive or twisting movements), opisthotonus, (spasm of the muscles causing backward arching of the head, neck and spine), trismus, (spasm of the jaw muscles causing the mouth to remain tightly closed), chorea, (a neurological disorder characterised by jerky involuntary movements affecting especially the shoulder, hips and face), and other dyskinesias, (abnormality or impairment of voluntary movement). Patients can also have prominent sialorrhea, (drooling or excessive salivation), dysarthria, (difficult or unclear articulation of speech that is otherwise linguistically normal), dysphasia, (difficulty swallowing).

Hyperthermia is a defining symptom according to many diagnostic criteria. Temperatures of more than 38 degree Celsius are typical, (87 %), but even higher temperatures, greater than 40 degree Celsius are common, (40 %).

Autonomic instability takes the form of tachycardia – excessive heart rate, (in 88 percent), labile or high blood pressure (in 61-77 percent) and tachyon – rapid breathing, (in 73 percent). Diaphoresis – sweating, is often profuse.

In an analysis of 340 cases, 70 % of patients followed a typical course of mental status changes appear first, followed by rigidity, then hyperthermia and autonomic dysfunction. Some case reports documented delay in the appearance of fever of more than 24 hours, leading to initial diagnostic confusion. There is substantial variability in the presentation of NMS, and other reports do not necessarily substantiate a typical course.

Laboratory Abnormalities:-

Elevated CK- creatine kinase. Laboratory findings often reflect the clinical manifestations of NMS with more severe rigidity leading to profound CK. Normal CK can be seen if rigidity is not clearly well developed, particularly early in the onset of the syndrome. Elevated CK, particularly in the mild to moderate range is not specific for NMS and is often seen in patients with acute and chronic psychosis due to intramuscular injections and physical restraints, and sometimes without specific explanation. CK levels greater than 1000 IU/L however, are probably more specific for NMS, and the degree of CK elevation correlates with disease severity and prognosis.

A case-controlled study demonstrated that patients with NMS were more likely to have elevated CK levels during previous non-NMS admissions than did controls, (76 versus 30 percent). CK levels do normalise after an NMS episode.

Other laboratory finding is leukocytosis, with white blood cell count typically 10,000 – 40,000/mm3. A left shift may be present.

Mild elevations of lactate dehydrogenase, alkaline phosphatase and liver transaminases are common.

Electrolyte abnormalities – hypocalcaemia, hypomagnesaemia, hypo and hyper anthemia, hyperaemia and metabolic acidosis are frequently observed.

Myoglobinuric acute renal failure can result from rhabdomyolysis.

A low serum iron concentration is commonly seen in NMS patients and is sensitive, (92 to 100 %), but not a specific marker for NMS among acutely ill psychiatric patients.

Atypical Cases.

There is debate in the literature about milder or atypical cases of NMS. A "forme fruste", of the syndrome has been suggested to occur in milder cases, those associated with lower potency agents, or those diagnosed early on. In particular, rigidity may be milder and perhaps even absent. Complicating this issue is the fact that the isolated appearance of dysautonomia, hyperthermia, Parkinsonism, rigidity and creatinase kinase elevations all occur with antipsychotic therapy. Individually they do not appear to be a harbinger of NMS. From a practical clinical point of view, it seems reasonable to consider diagnosis when any two of the tetrad of symptoms are present in the setting of an offending agent.

In patients with possible NMS, brain imaging studies and lumbar puncture are required to exclude structural brain disease and infection. MRI and CT scans are all typically normal. Cerebrospinal fluid is usually normal, but a non-specific elevation in protein is reported in 37 percent of cases.

Treatment.

Stop causative agent – removal of the causative agent is the single most important treatment in NMS. Other potential contributing psychotropic agents should also be stopped if possible.

Supportive care – The need for aggressive and supportive care in NMS is essential and uncontroversial. Complication are common and severe, even fatal. These include:-

Dehydration
Electrolyte imbalance
Acute renal failure associated with rhabdomyolysis
Cardiac arrythmias, including torsades de pointes and cardiac arrest.
Myocardial infarction
Cardiomyopathy
Respiratory failure from chest wall rigidity, aspiration pneumonia, pulmonary embolism.
Deep venous thrombophlebitis
Thrombocytopenia
Disseminated intravascular coagulation
Deep venous thrombosis
Hepatic failure
Sepsis.

The intensive nature of the required monitoring and supportive treatment are such that admission to the intensive care unit is required.

Residual catatonia can persist after other symptoms have resolved. Electroconvulsive therapy should be considered in those patients and those whom lethal catatonia is suspected, as an alternative or concomitant disorder“.

After reading various articles, I was convinced that my mother had suffered from NMS. Not only had I seen her with a lack of hydration, profuse sweating, increased muscle tone, extreme pallor, neck contortion, poking her tongue, stupor, mutism, immobility, poor nutritional intake, malnutrition, lack of balance; incontinence and body weight loss, but the doctors had no idea what the cause of these symptoms were.

I wrote my letter of complaint. It seemed rather inconsequential, considering the poor condition of my mother, but I felt my grievance had to be formal.

My letter was dated 26 August 2012 and was received by the Mental Health Unit on 02 September 2012:-

> "I am writing with reference to my mother Judith Allen who was originally admitted to Grianagh Court in October 2011, as an emergency admission, after my father had a stroke and went into hospital for some weeks. She had been on the waiting list for admission to yourselves for some time prior to this, I believe. I initially thought that I could cope with her at our home, but sadly I could only manage one week, due to her aggressive outbursts and severe mood swings.
>
> Since then, we have had one family meeting, which was prior to her leaving Grianagh Court to be admitted into Laxey Glen House Residential Home, which following her assessment was deemed to be suitable. Both myself and my father were aware that they were struggling with her towards the end of her stay there, and that they had asked for a meds review on a couple of occasions.
>
> My father then decided on Beaconsfield Home, where he believed that an E.M.I. unit was being set up. Regrettably, I was away on holiday at the time the decision was made. Again,

the staff expressed their concerns about the level of distress and agitation that my mother had. I believe that a review of meds and visits by Dr. Jagus were requested towards the end of her stay there, again. A couple of staff members informed us on how difficult they were finding coping with my mother's aggressive mood swings. A psychiatric male nurse told my father that Beaconsfield did not have the specialist staff or facilities to deal with her illness. With not being involved with the move to Beaconsfield, I am not aware if the Admission Team/ Management were informed on how extreme and disruptive she could be at times, which I feel should have been a major emphasis, to minimise the stress caused to my mother by moving yet again, (I presume a full report was requested and submitted by Laxey Glen House, the last Residential Home). This culminated in her eventual "section".

On going back to Grianagh Court, both my father and I felt that she was in the "best place", for reassessment.

In the last four months in Grianagh Court we have seen a decline in her health, both physically and mentally, and yet despite her unusual gait, she was still able to walk very well and could do so up and down the corridor there, for very long periods of time, occasionally breaking into a near run when my father visited. She could feed herself and drink for herself at this point too. In the previous week before her hospital admission, she peeled a banana for herself. (without prompting), and could eat it herself too. Presently she can barely move her arms and is not capable of scratching her own nose.

We have not been informed of her care plan or the medication prescribed to her, at any point, despite my father attending the unit every day.

In the two to three days prior to her hospital admission, we found her to be in a slumped, almost coma-like state. She was unable to sit-up by herself, let alone drink, feed or walk by herself. On visiting, we were told by various workers that her medication had been increased by Dr. Jagus, and that it would give her a well-needed rest. Cups of tea were made for her when we were there, but she was unable to drink them, even when we put them to her mouth, I informed staff of this and raised my concerns about her becoming dehydrated. My father raised his fears also. I reassured him that she was in the best place.

On visiting my mother with my husband, we emphasised our worries at her overly sedated state and the swelling around her face. We were told that a locum doctor was about to see her. When he visited, I underlined that my concerns about her state that coincided with the increase in medication. He in-turn informed me that he was only a "Community Doctor". Later that day, my father rang to say that my mother was being admitted to Noble's Hospital. I immediately went to see her at Grianagh Court, while she was waiting for the ambulance to transfer her. She was clearly dehydrated with crusted lips. And her neck and face were distinctly swollen. I tried to give her a drink, but she could not move her head without shrieking in pain. Her arms were also very rigid and swollen too.

At this point, I need to raise the question as to why staff were not monitoring her closely for reactions and interactions to her increased medication. Her face and neck were almost solid with swelling and her temperature was high, over 38, as witnessed when the Health Assistant took it.

When she was in Ward 2 a nurse said that they were concerned at her level of medication, as she was so sleepy – too drowsy to eat or drink. She could not be roused.

She was apparently sent back to Grianagh Court without a change in her medication, and without her resuming walking, eating, drinking, or any improvement in her level of sedation.

After her re-admission to Ward 4, I spoke with a doctor on Admissions and raised my concerns about her lack of mobility, eating/drinking and her general state of consciousness, which coincidentally happened since that increased levels of her medication at Grianagh Court.

At Ward 5. The Sister remarked on her concerns over the medication and in particular, she mentioned the length of time that my mother had been on risperidone, along with her levels of diazepam. This was the first time that I was made aware of the medication that she was taking.

On another occasion, I spoke with the doctor and explained how since the increased level of medication at Grianagh Court, my mother had lost her ability to walk, drink, or feed herself and was now in a coma-like state. I underlined that it may be coincidence, but that it did seem a little too coincidental. Why did no-one from Grianagh inform the hospital about her lack of mobility and lack of capacity to eat or drink earlier, all of which were lost within a day of being over-sedated.

On visiting my mother a few days later, and after her having M.R.I./C.T. scans and a lumbar puncture, all of which were apparently clear, the doctor informed me that all of her dementia drugs had now been stopped and that we should see an improvement in her over the next four days or so. It appeared that the medication was the likely cause, I was told. This was nearly four weeks after the increased dosage.

I am no medical professional, but in my lay experience, her sudden loss of ability to feed herself or drink, along with being immobile now, was something that happened far too suddenly and far too coincidentally. Was she ever checked for Neuroleptic Malignant Syndrome at any point? Did this not cross anybody's mind? She was taking three sedative drugs at the same time, one of which I believe was risperidone.

The levels of observation of her during the newly increased levels of medication appear to have been poor, along with the lack of ability to re-hydrate her, at a time when dehydration should have been avoided at all costs.

I personally feel that my father should have been informed as to the reasons why her levels of medication were being increased and that he should have been pre-warned about the state of her drowsiness that was to be expected in her. He was in Grianagh Court visiting her every day, barr a couple. Respect needs to be maintained towards the next of kin too. Lack of communication leads to high levels of frustration, along with feelings of helplessness and abandonment towards their loved ones.

Over the last ten months, we have experienced no stabilising of my mother's state. Where we had expected or hoped to see an easing of her agitation and distress, we have seen only an increase. Where we had hoped to find a settled, stable environment for her, we have found only continual disruption for her, proving stressful for all concerned.

In the physical state that we find my mother in at present, I do find myself wondering if the Older Persons Mental Health Unit has indeed failed her. People with mental health problems do seem to be at the bottom of the healthcare priorities agenda. I am hoping that this lack of care/diagnosis does not lead to my mother's needless death.

For future reference, I really do feel the need for my father to be kept informed of all my mother's medication prescribed, along with any changes to her medication too.

We do as a family appreciate the time and effort taken with my mother, but I also hope that you can see where our very serious concerns lay too.

Yours sincerely
Victoria Quine"

16
Salvage Operation

The good news was that Judith was now to remain in Ward 5. We had no idea who had made that final decision, but we were thankful, as the level of care that she was receiving appeared to surmount any that she had previously.

While visiting my mother, the Sister came over to me for a chat, during which time, I explained that I was unhappy with the care that she had received from the Consultant Psychiatrist and from the unit itself. The risperidone prescribed to Judith, should have been relayed to my father and myself along with the risks to Judith's health associated with this drug, explained to us. The Mental Health Services seemed to act of their own accord. I was upset over this, I explained. I went on to inform her that I had written a letter of complaint to the Mental Health Unit. She advised me to write the complaint to the main hospital, as Grianagh Court and the Mental Health Services, were a, "law unto themselves", and advised me that my complaint would be, "swept under the carpet", as such. She then handed me a "Complaint Leaflet", detailing the formal complaint procedure. I perused the pamphlet and noted that Mental Health Services complaints should be directed to them. She advised me to boycott that route.

Worryingly, Judith continuously kept dislodging her N.G. tube, and she was still refusing anything more than one spoonful of food, at any one time. My father, myself and Nigel were to attend a meeting with various Consultants, including the Old Age Psychiatrist, Dr. Jagus; Dr Majeed, who had worked with my mother's condition closely and Consultant Dr Balakrishnan. This meeting was to be held at Noble's hospital on 07 September, 2012. There was no substantial change in Judith's presentation. She had become more responsive and a little more vocal – occasional words were coherent, but mainly the word, "no".

My father expressed concern whilst in the ward one day. He complained that two male healthcare assistants should not be addressing Judith's incontinence needs. He was quite angry. In hindsight, this should not have been allowed. A patient's dignity should still be respected, no matter how incapacitated they appear to be. I had also been unsettled by the fact that the Mental Health unit had packed up all of Judith belongings from the unit, into a clear dustbin liner and deposited it beside her hospital bed without informing us. It had niggled me but seemed insignificant in the great scheme of things. The bigger picture was so much graver. It was becoming crystal clear by now, that Judith would never regain her mobility or speech, and the doctors had no explanation for her condition. I so hoped that I was wrong, but I felt sure that my mother would indeed die from her condition. Dr. Majeed had informed me already, that medically, there was nothing more they could do for Judith.

The meeting for the 07 September, 2012, was upon us. I was physically nervous. I had so many questions that I wished to ask, but I would probably forget to ask, as I am not an articulate person in strange circumstances, but I was determined to do the very best available to me. I had written questions that I wanted to present in the meeting, in a notebook for ease of reference, but I knew under pressure, and in the strange environment, with new people, that I would struggle with being nervous and uncomfortable.

I wished for a split second that I could ring in, "sick", but I told myself I had to be strong – that I was strong.

Walking from the car park to the hospital made me feel nauseous. My legs were trembling and the cold wind battering my face, offered no relief. This soon diminished when I met my father in the hospital entrance. He was so very frail, drawn and grey. He spoke in a flat, monotone manner, like he had lost the will to live. We hugged and I tried my utmost not to become emotional. The tears I managed to stifle, rerouted themselves down my nose. I needed to quickly buy some paper handkerchiefs from the shop, along with a bottle of water. My nerves always made my mouth as arid as a desert, and my tongue would get sandwiched to my palate. I was wishing the day over, before it had even really begun.

We entered a boardroom, with a large round table, with plain greyish blue upholstered chairs scattered around it. Some doctors were already sitting; others arrived a few minutes later. Dr. Jagus and Dr. Majeed I recognised and knew. Others just by facial recognition; others I did not know.

At the beginning of the meeting, I asked all present if they objected to me recording the meeting. All agreed to this.

Dr. Majeed opened the meeting.

This is a partial transcript of that meeting:-

Dr Majeed, "Do you want to know the medical history of what we've been doing so far?"

Me, "Absolutely, yes".

Dr Majeed, "Initially when she came in, she was treated by the surgical team for possible pyelonephritis, as an infection of the kidneys, probably. When she came to us, we were treating her for possible cholecystitis, inflammation of the gallbladder. Subsequently, we thought she might have an underlying encephalitis, inflammation and infection of the brain basically, so we treated her for that with fourteen days of antibiotics and anti-viral medication. In the meantime, she had a few scans. She had an ultrasound scan which showed she had a big stone sitting in the gallbladder. The CT scan didn't show much apart from the fact that she had previous changes to her brain because of the age related, basically. She had blood cultures came back positive. I'm not exactly sure for what organism, but she had been treated for that anyway. She had E-coli in the past and that's been treated. I think that's pretty much it. That's where we stand at the moment, and obviously issues at the moment are mobility. She stills remains drowsy and feeding. These are the three main issues we have at the moment.

Me, "Okay, do we know what the cause may be for the not eating?

Dr Majeed, "From the medical point of view, we have kind of, as such, covered all the aspects for her.......we initially were thinking about infections and treating all those things, which we have done already. I don't think there is anything from the medical point of view that will cause her to be that drowsy the way she is, basically, so it's more.....I don't think it's ... we have treated all possible causes we were thinking of, in her particular case".

Me, "Sure. From our point of view, when we came to Grianagh Court, the major, major problem that we saw was the swelling in the neck. It was huge swelling. And the arms as well were swollen. It was a bizarre thing that I've never seen before".

Dr Jagus, "Just prior to coming here?".

Me: "Yes, from Grianagh Court. I can give you a full actual breakdown of what happened. We actually mentioned to the nurse in Grianagh Court, that we weren't happy with the level of sedation, and she was literally in a coma kind of state. We also said that we were concerned about her not being able to drink anything and we thought that she may become dehydrated., which she did become when she was taken into Ward 2. On each case in Ward 2 and Ward 4, I highlighted the fact of this solid, absolutely solid, swelling in her neck. It was just so solid, and her arms were just so solid. She couldn't move her neck. Margaret Quayle (should have been Halsall), from Grianagh Court, I specifically raised this. We saw a doctor who came to see her before she was admitted, again raised it with him. Later on, Dad rang and said that she was being admitted because you were concerned in Grianagh Court about her. She went into Ward 2. Again, we said that we were concerned about her lack of movement, her lack of eating, the consciousness. When she was released from Ward 2, they said that they weren't aware of the issues with not being able to eat, not being able to walk that she had lost whilst she was in Grianagh Court. That's where our concern was, on that level. As a little bit of research that we've done afterwards, we wondered whether it might be that Neuroleptic Malignant Syndrome that was there. She was on three lots of neuroleptic drugs at that time. And this coma like state that she was in, was our major concern......"

Dr Jagus interrupts, "She also had Pyelonephritis. She had a severe renal infection which......"

Me, "Sure, sure...."

My father, "Somebody did say at Grianagh Court that you had doubled the dose of her medicine and then they said that they would have to put it down to what is was before".

Dr Jagus, "I think when I look back, she was seen by ......I'm just trying to think back....I was just looking through the notes before I came down. Dr. O'Sullivan, who was there at the time, did pop her risperidone up to 1mg at the time, but I think the significant change both in mental state and mobility etc., is tied in with Pyelonephritis. I think....I've seen it in people who have got slight dementia, that any even minor infections can cause a very major change. It's a very significant infection Pyelonephritis, because she required I.V. antibiotics which is essentially why we were also concerned about her physical state which is why she came over here to have that treated and then it was very, very clear that even when that was treated she was still physically unwell and there was something else. Hence further investigation. She did briefly come back to us?

Me, "She did".

Dr. Jagus, "She came back to us because that had been treated, but we still had problems with poor function and increased confusion. We know that she suffers with significant impairment and cognition, but it was still much more significant than usual".

Me, "When she came back from Ward 2 to Grianagh Court she still had this solid swelling".

Dr Jagus, "And still physically unwell, poor diet, poor mobility".

Me, "No consciousness at all".

Dr Jagus, "And it was the gall bladder this time – whether it ties in, I don't know, but it was certainly one infection after another. She's got quite a big gallstone, hasn't she?"

Dr Majeed, "30mm. Significant – I think in seven years it is the first one that I have seen that big".

Dr Jagus, "I actually came to see her over here whilst she was in the midst of that treatment. It was quite clear that she was still kind of semi-conscious, had a drip up and wasn't eating or drinking at that stage. I don't think she was taking oral medication at that point either, and obviously along with that, that meant that she wasn't taking any of the sedative medication she had, and also right through that period when she had been drowsy for some reason, she hadn't been taking them then, either – what that drowsiness was I'm not quite sure, but it was understandable that you would want to screen her for encephalitis".

(It is important to highlight at this point of the transcript that Judith's medical history, detailed that Dr Jagus had in fact visited the ward in question, and due to her drowsiness, Dr Jagus instructed the discontinuation of her Pregablin medication and her Risperidone on 31 July, 2012, 2 days after she was admitted to this ward. Dr Jagus reduced her diazepam, from 5mgs to 2mgs three times a day. He instructed that she was still to continue with the Sodium Valproate 100mgs three times a day. On 20 August 2012, Dr Jagus instructed a gradual reduction of Sodium Valproate by 100mgs each dose time. This makes his above statement totally untrue).

Dr Majeed, "From the medical point of view, we've done extensive runs of blood test, scans and everything including lumbar puncture – it was quite difficult, because she was drowsy, and needed two members of staff and three of us to actually do the lumbar puncture. Unfortunately, as Dr Jagus said, from a medical point of view, I can't really explain why, you know".

Me, "Is it possible that she had Neuroleptic Malignant Syndrome?".

Dr Jagus, "It's possible, but – it's possible, but I think because .... Unlikely, and the fact that at that point the neuroleptics would have been stopped. She's not taking them and wouldn't have been taking them anyway, and.".

Me, "Sure, but it's just...."

Dr Jagus, "Yes, Yes, I understand".

Me, "It just seems too coincidental".

Dr Jagus, "I know .... Perhaps what ..... just think retrospectively, I haven't got the benefit of the notes in front of me, I suspect what might have happened – don't quote me on that – the medication, because she was developing something like that, there may have been a change in her behavioural symptoms, agitation – as you know she's been very distressed. Whether it was felt appropriate to increase it at that stage – it's difficult to know – you can't pin these things down. I can understand your concerns about it".

Me, "She was clearly dehydrated when she went into Ward 2".

Dr Jagus, "I think what can tie in at that stage, is that physically we were concerned that there was something else – an infection and her temperature was raised, and it was clear when she got here that it was renal tract".

Me, "The strange thing is that when we went into Ward 2 and we spoke with the doctor, he said that, about the Cholecystitis, that they weren't worried about it and weren't going to operate or take it any further, so at this point how serious was this infection to not take it any further?".

Dr Majeed, "The thing is from the Cholecystitis point of view there are two schools of thought. One is somebody comes in with Cholecystitis, some Consultant will take them straight down to theatre and take the gall bladder out. For forty eight hours they will stay on antibiotics – for a week, or ten days, however long it takes them to recover. They recover – they go home. Other school of thought is, a lot of Consultants don't operate on a hot gall bladder. What they do is sit on it, give them antibiotics, make them better. In three or four months' time, see them as an outpatient and see what symptoms they are getting. If they are getting better then as a plan, they go for elective surgery. They don't rush in and do the surgery, so from a surgical point of view I wouldn't be able to comment, but these are the two different schools of thought, that is normal to be seen in practice, basically".

Jim, "When was Judy taken of all her medications? I am sure that one of the doctors said that she was going to be taken off all her medication".

Dr Jagus, "There was a significant period of time when she wasn't able to take anything".

Jim, "Because when this doctor told me that she had been taken off all of her medication, she improved, greatly hasn't she? (Father looks towards me). She was awake and was beginning to speak even. This was after I was told....".

Dr Jagus, "She's much better now".

Jim, "Sorry?".

Dr Jagus, "I mean, when I saw her a few days ago, when I came to see her, she was quite clearly very different to when I'd seen her before".

Jim, "She's improved a lot in the last week".

Further on in the meeting:-

Me, "Is it possible that she has Schizophrenia or something?

Dr Jagus, "No, as you know with your mum, it has been a long and difficult case as she's so young, but it is clear that **she's got very early.......well, not very early, but early and rapidly progressing dementia".**

Me: Is it dementia caused by Alzheimer's".

Dr. Jagus, "Alzheimer's is just the commonest form of dementia. People often think of Alzheimer's disease as something else, but it is just the name for the commonest type. At the beginning we thought, when she first came, if you can remember, we thought that it was depression at first, but there was something not quite right about it. She was very depressed at the beginning – we treated that and that improved, but she was left with these beginning of this memory impairment which has progressed ever since".

Me: "Right, it just appears that she is hallucinating".

Dr Jagus, "Which again can be very much part of the picture of dementia. People think it's just a problem with memory, but you get so many other symptoms, like confusion, hallucinations, agitation, often. You were having problems with her at home getting quite aggressive – there was a big personality change.

Jim, "Yes".

Dr Jagus, "but in terms of the overall picture over the last four years is it, three, or maybe four years, the pattern is really what you would expect to find with patients who come to me when they are younger. I've watched them become a bit more aggressive quicker, and then you add things in on top of that like infections, particularly significant infections like this one, you often see a huge change in not only their mental state, but their physical state, like mobility and eating".

This is not exhaustive of the transcription from the meeting. We went on to discuss dementia in further detail. During the meeting I asked Dr Jagus if they would consider ECT, (electroconvulsive therapy), on my mother. He informed me that Judith was not strong enough and it was not a consideration.

ECT has proved to be successful in treating residual catatonic signs after NMS. (ref. Caroff SN, et al. J Clin Psychopharmacol 2000).

The "improvement over the last week", that my father mentioned in the meeting, was after the Sodium Valproate was the final medication to be stopped. Sodium Valproate is now known to precipitate NMS especially when used with antipsychotic drugs concurrently, which it had been for over eleven days, whilst Judith was admitted to the medical wards at the hospital.

(ref www.ncbi.nlm.nih.gov/pmc/articles/PMC5290716) (ref Clinical Psychopharmacology and Neuroscience 2017 Feb: 15 (1): 76-78 Author Veli Yilidrim et al),

The first time that Judith met with Dr Jagus was in 2008. For her anxiety due to depression Pregablin, (Lyrica), had been prescribed and Mirtazapine for the depression itself. Mirtazapine like other medications that affect serotonin can cause a potentially fatal syndrome known as neuroleptic malignant syndrome. Mirtazapine is known as a tetracyclic antidepressant. (ref: Druglib.com). Risk for potentially life-threatening serotonin syndrome and neuroleptic malignant syndrome-like reactions has been reported with SSRIs, SNRI's MAOIs, and other serotonergic drugs used as immunotherapy, but particularly with concomitant use of the following the following agents: serotonergic drugs (including triptans), drugs that impair metabolism of serotonin, antipsychotic (Risperidone is classed as), dopamine antagonists, and non-psychiatric MAOIs. (rxlist.com Medical ad Pharmacy Editor: John P Cunha, DO, FACOEP).

Mirtazapine has also been reported to cause rhabdomyolysis – muscle wasting.

Judith had also been taking donezepil, (Aricept) a dementia drug, for some considerable time and during her stay in the medical ward, and this is also known to induce Neuroleptic Malignant Syndrome.

(ref: International Journal of Neuropsychopharmacology, Volume 7, Issue 1, March 2004. Neuroleptic malignant syndrome induced by donezepil. Author T Matsumoto et al)

The Government of Canada issued new warnings in 2015, for the Alzheimer's drug Aricept (donezepil) advising of the risk of two rare but potentially serious conditions: muscle breakdown (rhabdomyolysis) and a neurological disorder called neuroleptic malignant syndrome (NMS). (www.healthycanadians.gc.ca/recall-alert-rappel-avis/hc-sc/2015/43469a-eng.php

17

The Balance Sheet

Following the meeting, I was very confused. Things just did not make sense to me. Why had the two Sisters on Ward 5 mentioned their concerns over the risperidone medication, if it was not still being administered to Judith? How would they know about prior medication and why would they jeopardise their positions in order to raise this matter?

My mother had been in a Mental Health Unit accredited by the Royal College of Psychiatrists, as being in the top ten per cent of the best units in the UK – accredited not just once, but twice.

I found that I was doubting myself. Was I being overly cautious, or was I being, "spectrum special?" I was torn between feeling like an out-and-out troublemaker and being downright certain that the unusual condition that I had witnessed in my mother, was Neuroleptic Malignant Syndrome. It was like a tug of war, between sadness, anxiety and hope together, competing against will and determination, to find the crux of what was going on. I would do whatever was humanly possible to get to the root of this phenomenon. Nothing would stop me – not my husband, not lack of any finance. I would go through the motions at the very least to hear all perspectives on this condition. My hopes for my mother were waning, but my determination to ensure this never happened to another person was all consuming and intense. I sensed that a major injustice had been done early on. My mother, as difficult as she could be, still had a right to life. The Mental Health Services seemed to be treating her with utter disdain. No caution at all had been exercised, when prescribing Judith's medication.

Clearly, Dr Jagus displayed this lack of concern by explaining that Alzheimer's was just the most common form of dementia.

In the meeting on 07 September, I had turned to see a "stern glance", from Dr Jagus towards Dr Majeed. This made me realise that this was not a, "cosy, informal meeting". Behind the scenes I suspected that there was more to it. Noble's Hospital had an ongoing lack of confidence surrounding it. To the extent that the West Midlands Quality Review Service were called in to evaluate the hospitals performance and investigate subsequent findings. They were commissioned to undertake this by The Isle of Man Department of Health and Social Care, to perform a rolling programme of external independent quality assurance reviews of the Island's health service between 2013 and 2018. Two Chief Executives had left recently – one on rather early retirement, the other on resignation. More politicians were voicing their concerns, and disconcertingly, ten doctors had signed an, "open letter", expressing their concerns too. Since 2012 there have been a plethora of Chief Executives who have either retired early or resigned.

I seriously hoped that my mother was not going to be a victim of such intimidating circumstances and failures.

During the meeting on 07 September, it had been discussed that Judith might benefit from having a PEG, (percutaneous endoscopic gastrostomy), which is a medical procedure in which a tube is passed into a patient's stomach through the abdominal wall to provide means of feeding, when oral intake is not sufficient. This was suggested, as Judith was constantly dislodging the NG tube. My father and I both needed to think long and hard about this option. It was something that we never expected to be addressing. Certainly, not at this present time.

My mother's on-going Care Worker, Marie had been present in the meeting, but had just observed. She later rang me in the evening to see how I thought the meeting had gone. I played my cards very close to my chest. She then went on to ask if I had noticed her cold sores on her mouth, in a chirpy way, as if we were best of buddies. I informed her that Compeed was normally very good. Yet it appeared to me that she had undergone a lip filler procedure, that looked to have gone wrong, or that she had taken a reaction to. I guessed she had rung solely to gauge my reactions to the meeting.

For the next few days, both myself and my father visited Judith daily. Some days she would just sleep, and on other days she would be fretful and tearful. Occasional words were now audible from Judith. The majority of which were, "No", "Yes", "Help", "Mummy", and, "Jim". Whilst still incredibly disturbing to see her incapacitated and bed-bound, any slight improvement was a giant step in the right direction.

Dr Jagus re-prescribed Mirtazapine to Judith, to encourage her appetite. To us, as a family, it was a point-blank refusal of Judith to eat that we were seeing, and she would become angry or frightened at the mere sight of food.

The reply to my letter of complaint to the Mental Health Unit eventually arrived, dated 19 September, 2012:-

> "Dear Mrs V Quine
> Thank you for your letter dated 26 August, 2012.
>
> I have investigated your complaints and discussed the issues with Dr Jagus, he informed me of the family meeting held at Noble's Hospital Re Judith, and some of your concerns may have been addressed and resolved.
>
> I understand the concerns you have expressed about your mother's care whilst a patient at Grianagh Court. Having reviewed the documentation, I have found the nursing staff on Grianagh Court did monitor and care for Judith at all times and especially any side effects of medication. This was evidenced in the notes and communication with medication staff. Mr Allen visited every day and was updated by staff on duty.

If you still have any concerns, please do not hesitate to contact me and I will arrange a meeting with Dr. Jagus and myself.

Yours sincerely
Mrs Doreen Fell
Senior Practitioner
Ward Manager"

Firstly, the meeting on 07 September, 2012, addressed very little of my concerns and had in fact raised more additional questions. Secondly, when I was in Grianagh Court and asked to see Judith's "obs", the nurse told me that they didn't undertake daily vital observations. Thirdly, as for updating my father, he knew nothing about the medication being prescribed to Judith. It had never been discussed with him.

This letter I considered to be a, "fob-off".

Despite the poorly condition of my mother and the strain that we were all feeling, I felt compelled to write the letter of complaint to the main hospital itself, as the Sister on Ward 5 had recommended. Hopefully somebody might take this matter seriously.

At this point I knew nothing about the young man, Ben Hall, 25, who had died at the unit, just weeks before my mother was admitted to hospital for the first time from Grianagh Court. His death was due to ligature strangulation, whilst feeling suicidal in Grianagh Court. He was found to have died as a result of gross systemic failure on the part of the Department of Health, when he hung himself from a non-collapsible shower rail. Worryingly, the computer with the relevant files had been wiped, leading the Coroner to question whether reports had been completed in the manner expected. Most disturbingly, the Coroner John Needham found, "if basic medical care had been provided in the way expected it was more likely than not that Mr Hall would not have died as he did. Equally concerning, is the fact that this was a Royal College of Psychiatrists "accredited", mental health unit.

I sat down alone, later that night and compiled my letter. As a lay-person, my knowledge was limited at this point, but I had plenty of commitment and conviction to this situation. I had no access to medical records at this point, but I was certain that my mother had suffered from Neuroleptic Malignant Syndrome.

18

The Irreparable Damage

Judith's physical condition appeared to be deteriorating due to her refusal to eat and the continual dislodging of the NG tube and on the 13 September, 2012, Judith was refusing the renewal of the NG tube too.

My father and I spoke with Dr Majeed, who advised that the time had come, when we, as the next of kin, needed to make a decision about Judith having a PEG inserted, enabling direct feeding into the stomach. We could not hesitate with this option, as we could see no other alternative available. The procedure for fitting the PEG was scheduled for 18th September; however, this was postponed until 20 September due to Judith's low potassium levels; replacement therapy was commenced. We were hopeful that this PEG would provide at least the nutrients that Judith required. The dietician had assessed my mother previously and stated that there were no problems with Judith swallowing. Judith's point-blank refusal to eat was most concerning and frustrating.

Judith had the PEG inserted on 21 September, 2012. There were complications with the operation, when my mother had stopped breathing for nearly ten minutes under general anaesthetic. We were unaware of this at the time. We had been worried about Judith going under anaesthetic due to her poor physical condition, but due to her agitated manner, local anaesthetic was probably not an option. When we saw her back in the ward after the fitting of the PEG, she seemed rather upbeat and generally happy, despite the circumstances and the trauma involved.

The nurse explained to my father and myself, that a feeding regime would start, although it had to be a slow, gradual process, as it could be dangerous to commence her on too much nutritional intake immediately. The PEG was administered with nutrition, fluid and medication by nursing staff, but after two days Judith was vomiting and in pain. The stoma was seen to be distended and the area was leaking. Investigations were needed.

A PR (per rectum), was done, (as noted by the doctor), but done in a difficult position as Judith was unable to flex/bend her legs towards her chest. (A sign of rigidity). X-rays showed no obstruction in the PEG. Her heart rate and blood pressure were raised, and her temperature was 35.5 degrees Celsius. Her extremities were noted as being cold.

Judith was nil by PEG from 23 September.

On 26 September, as noted in medical records, Judith shouted, "Help", to nursing staff. They immediately came and noted blood coming for the PEG. Upon a doctor examining her, cellulitis was observed around the wound, with slight leakage. Judith was crying when they flushed the PEG with water. Judith began projectile vomiting brown foul-smelling fluid. She was noted as cold and clammy. I.V. fluids were started. Faecal matter around the PEG suggested perforated bowel. Judith was actually vomiting faecal matter. It was suggested that Judith had dislodged the PEG from her stomach. Judith was wrapped in silver hypothermic blankets.

Dr Majeed spoke with me and my husband during our evening visit to my mother. He explained that Judith would possibly go into multi-organ failure. He asked me to consent with a, "Do not resuscitate order". I consented – Judith's quality of life was now beyond torturous. A PICC line was inserted into her arms and her pyjama top was to cover it, to prevent dislodgement.

On 29 September, the PEG site dressing was removed, with a thick, foul-smelling green fluid oozing from it. When the abdomen was pressed, more green fluid emerged. The PEG was left on free drainage. The wound was cleaned, and a new dressing applied. This day should have been a day for celebration. It was Judith's 70th birthday. We had, so, so, hoped for good news and celebration. It was not to be.

On 01 October, 2012, Dr Krishnan met with my father, my husband and myself to explain that surgeons were concerned about reinserting the PEG into Judith's stomach. They believed that the risks to her, outweighed the benefits, and infection along with pain was highly likely, as Judith was likely to remove or dislodge the PEG with her recent renewed movement of her arms. My mother refused to eat, and despite Dr. Jagus insisting on re-introducing Mirtazapine medication which might increase her appetite, it had not been successful. She was reluctant to take anything orally. All options had been attempted yet had failed.

Later on, Dr Majeed arranged for a meeting for the next day at the hospital. It was decided that Judith should be allowed to pass away under the Liverpool Care Pathway – palliative care. No artificial feeding or I.V. fluids would be administered. The patient would be refused the basic requirements for life to continue. We were passed on a lever-arch file that would explain the process. Both my father and I were dumbfounded. We perused the file, but nothing registered with us. Just a sense of shock. We were informed that medically there was nothing more they could do or provide to Judith. We could attempt to feed her, but if she refused, then nature would take its course.

It was a decision made with no viable alternative option, that we could see either.

My research on Neuroleptic Malignant Syndrome did not provide an answer either. Early recognition of the disease and discontinuation of the NMS inducing medication, were the most crucial starting points to halting it. These were the only two things that would reduce mortality. Neither of these happened, despite false statements that the drugs had been stopped/not taken upon admission, by Dr Jagus, and Dr Tim Byrne.

My poor father. I had to steady him with my arm around his waist, as his legs swooned beneath him. He was a man of few words, but he said, "That bloody unit has done this to my Judy". I said nothing and remained silent. I felt trapped in a nightmare. Looking at my father's ashen, angry face, made me wonder how much more could he take. The sadness and cruelty of the situation was turning my stomach. I beckoned my father to sit in the chair near to him and I signalled for Nigel to stay with him. I proceeded to the bathroom just in time to throw-up. Tears rolled down my face – I wanted to not be an adult at that moment. Yet I knew I had to be strong to support my father. I splashed my face with cold tap water and dabbed at it with a paper towel, removing my smudged black eyeliner. I gave myself a lick of lipstick and exited the washroom; stepping back into reality.

My father was sitting with his head in his hands. Nigel was with his arm around Jim's shoulder. There was no conversation. Nothing to say. We were just too numb; reeling from the shocking news. My thoughts were jumping from one issue to another. Backwards and forwards; to and fro. Surely we could entice my mother to eat. She must want to eat her favourite food. Big cake with fresh cream. Trifle, yoghurt, walnuts, sweets ......just anything to keep her alive.

I asked my father to stay over at our house, but he declined. He wanted to go to bed at his house. I felt like my head was going to short-circuit. I didn't even have the energy to reason, or further persuade him. He looked totally emotionless now, drained of the will to keep going. We all had a lot to fathom our heads around.

I waited until the following day to explain the situation to my daughter, Sophie. When I did, she was understandably, equally devastated.

Later, I composed my letter of complaint, using the limited knowledge that I had since my research on Neuroleptic Malignant Syndrome. The letter could have been better, but I was armed with the limited facts and no access to the medical notes of my mother's at that point:-

"Dear Sir/Madam
I am writing to you with regards to my mother, Judith Allen, d.o.b. 29 September 1942, who was admitted to Nobel's Hospital on 20 July, 2012, from Grianagh Court's Elderly Persons Unit.

I wish to make a complaint that Dr. Jagus and Grianagh Court have failed in their duty of care towards my mother. They missed symptoms of Neuroleptic Malignant Syndrome and allowed her to become dehydrated, which should have been avoided at all costs, considering the medications that she was on. Dr. Jagus, I believe, has failed in his duty to ensure that she was treated for Neuroleptic Malignant Syndrome, alongside the infections that she was admitted to hospital for. He should have raised the issue upon her admission. He knew the exceptionally high risk that the drugs he was prescribing put her at but chose to ignore this. As a top Elderly Psychiatrist, it is impossible for him not to have known the risk associated. Urine infections and other infections can be a direct symptom of Neuroleptic Malignant Syndrome.

Prior to her admission to Noble's, I had witnessed an unusual muscle gain on my mother's legs when I changed her after she wet herself, in Grianagh Court on 30 May, 2012. I put this down to her excessive pacing of the corridor. It was such a noticeable change in muscle bulk, that I commented on it to my husband, and remarked that she now had legs like a professional footballer. I now believe that this change was a direct symptom of her developing Neuroleptic Malignant Syndrome.

Dr Jagus was prescribing Diazepam, Risperidone and Mirtazapine together, which culminated in her being left in a coma-like state for days, before being admitted to Noble's. Surely three lots of Neuroleptic drugs should give concern for the highest possible levels of monitoring of my mother.

Myself and my father commented on her state to the Grianagh Court staff, who said that her medication levels had been increased and that it was for her own good and would give her a well-needed rest. We raised the issue of our concerns about her becoming dehydrated. A condition that I now know should have been avoided at all costs, whilst being prescribed risperidone.

Neither my father or me were aware of the drugs that she was taking, or of the high risks associated with elderly dementia patients taking risperidone. I believe that the licensing of risperidone recommends short-term use of it for six weeks only, when treating aggression in dementia patients. I believe that my mother has been prescribed it for a lot longer. Risperidone is an antipsychotic drug linked to Neuroleptic Malignant Syndrome. I find it a very careless attitude to prescribe it, as it has been to my mother, without serious checks being done regularly. What checks have been made over the course of prescribing it to my mother?

She developed a shuffling gait whilst a Grianagh Court, which I now know can be a symptom of Neuroleptic Malignant Syndrome. She became doubly incontinent – another symptom of it.

I believe that there was a significant change in her level of aggression and agitation prior to her admission to Noble's Hospital – I believe another sign of developing NMS. This resulted in her levels of risperidone being increased, along with her diazepam. Changing her levels in this antipsychotic can trigger an episode too, or further enhance it.

I therefore believe that Grianagh Court's Elderly Persons Unit were not monitoring her closely enough and that Dr. Jagus should have ensured that the Neuroleptic drugs were to be withdrawn and treatment for Neuroleptic Malignant Syndrome should have ran alongside any treatment for infection. He of all people should know of the possible fatal consequences of not treating this condition. I believe that he has failed in his duty to my mother, and I wonder how many other patients may have been fatally failed, and how many will be in the future.

I believe that failure to treat her for NMS has resulted in her becoming bedridden due to severe muscle necrosis – a direct symptom of it, that should have been treated. Failure to treat this results in the highest mortality rates among sufferers.

I believe that she was left in a residual catatonic state, (a direct result of NMS), which can result in refusal to eat and a balance problem. This can last for weeks or even months.

Two of the doctors on Ward 5 have said that Neuroleptic Malignant Syndrome was a consideration, when pressed. Dr Jagus himself admitted that there was a possibility, when in a meeting on Ward 5 on 07 September.

My mother is currently being allowed to pass away under the Liverpool Care Pathway following the unsuccessful fitting of PEG feeding tube. I believe that her death will be a direct result in failures in duty by both Grianagh Court Elderly Persons Unit and Dr. Jagus.

I have enclosed my first letter of concern sent to Grianagh Court Elderly Persons Unit, for your information. I look forward to your response to my concerns.

Yours faithfully
Victoria Quine"

19

Helpless

The next day at the Ward, my father was already with Judith. The room had been decorated with two posies of flowers. Judith was thankfully on I.V. fluids still.

In desperation, Jim had done exactly as I had thought of doing and had brought in different items of Judith's favourite food. At first it seemed to be working. My father placed a completely ripped open bag of crisps on her over-bed table in front of her. She managed to grab and eat about five crisps, but she then stopped. He challenged her further with various foods; strawberry trifle; chocolate cookies; cheese cubes; salad; walnuts; banana and a selection of sweets. She refused any further food. I attempted with items that I had brought, but with no further success. Judy was raging by now. My father was frustrated and started talking loudly to Judith, pleading with her to eat. This made her agitated and angry. She began to shout back at Jim. Some of her words were inaudible, but, "fucking", was perfectly coherent, a number of times. It was so unusual for my mother normally, as I had never in my life heard her swear like that, prior to her present condition. If it wasn't so sad, it may have been amusing.

My father left the ward for a while following this. It was all too much for him. I suspected he had gone to smoke a cigar. He had given up for a number of years, but I guessed he was getting a little relief from the extreme stress of events.

One of the regular nurses came in to check on Judith. She had a sympathetic smile and was very gentle in her approach with us.

Jim returned and asked the nurse if he could bring some C.D.s and a C.D player in for Judy and he continued to explain how she had loved music and dancing. The nurse informed him that he could bring anything in that he wished to, if he thought it would make her more comfortable. He smiled, and I assumed he was already thinking about the music that she would like.

We sat there in the private room that Judith now had. She was rambling and making no sense, but the words were clearer than they had been since she arrived in the hospital. She still could not sit up straight and we often had to prop her up to make her look more comfortable. She was on an inflatable mattress which seemed to be continually inflating and deflating, I presumed to stop any pressure sores. Judith had now been bed-bound for nearly three months. Her weight had plummeted, yet her skin looked amazing, with hardly a line on her face. Many of the nurses commented that she never looked seventy years of age. She had the skin of a thirty five year old, one nurse had said. Still I couldn't believe that my mother would soon die, after all she had fought off, whilst in hospital. The anorexia was going to get the better of her.

I received a letter from Noble's Hospital on 18 October, 2012, but dated 09 October, 2012.:-

> "Dear Mrs Quine
> Thank you for your letter dated 04 October 2012 received in this office 5 October 2012. I am sorry that you have had cause to complain about the service we provide and will investigate your concerns under Local Resolution of the Isle of Man NHS Complaints Procedure.
>
> It is our normal practice, by reason of confidentiality, to obtain the patient's consent before we investigate a complaint made by a third party. This will indicate that your mother, Mrs Judith Allen is happy for you to act upon her behalf and that she consents to the release of the details of the investigation to you. However, on this occasion, consent will be waived.

As part of our procedures, I would like to offer you a meeting early in the process, upon receipt of consent, to see if we can bring about an early resolution to some, if not all, of your concerns and the issues you have identified. If you think this would be useful, could you telephone this office on 650792 and speak with my secretary, Jan, who will arrange this for you. You may, of course, be accompanied at this meeting. It would be my intention to arrange to meet with the most appropriate senior manager and/clinician that can help in your case. If I have not heard from you within five working days from the date of our letter, I will assume you do not want a meeting at this particular time and I will continue to investigate your concerns and forward a formal response once completed.

In line with Local Resolution of the Isle of Man NHS Complaint procedure, our aim is to respond to your complaint within 20 working days following receipt of consent. However, there are, unfortunately, some instances when we are unable to achieve these time scales, either due to the complexity of the complaint which can involve more than one department, or a member of staff involved in the investigation is absent from work. If there is a delay, I will keep you informed.

I have enclosed a Patient's Guide, which I hope you will find helpful.

Yours sincerely
Antony P R Warham (Patient Safety and Governance Manager)"

When I rang the office and spoke with Amanda Mills, to arrange a meeting, I was informed that the window of opportunity for a meeting had now passed.

I explained that the letter had not arrived until that day, and I could send a photo of the post-mark if she so wished.

She informed me that she would attempt to arrange a meeting, and would confirm by letter, the date and time.

The next day, the letter arrived informing me of the meeting.

"Dear Mrs Quine
Further to my telephone conversation with you on 18 October 2012, may I please advise that I have arranged for you to meet with Dr Tim Byrne, Clinical Director, Mental Health Services, Mr Steve Chell, Head of Mental Health Services, Dr Balakrishnan, Consultant Physician and I on Thursday 25 October at 4.00pm.

The meeting will be held in the Small Meeting Room, Management Suite, Noble's Hospital. If, on arrival, you inquire at Reception in the Main Entrance to Noble's Hospital, you will be assisted with directions.

Yours sincerely
Amanda Mills
Case Manager
Patient Safety and Governance".

20
The Death Toll

The next few days were very similar to the previous days. Judith was still on I.V.fluids, and remained consistent in refusing any food, except the occasional spoonful of yoghurt. Despite this, her mood was cheery now, and she was even singing along to a Daniel O'Donnell C.D., that my father brought in. Even the nurses noted the singing in Judith's medical records. We constantly tried to encourage Judith to eat every visiting time. It was truly upsetting when she declined all offerings.

The hospital had arranged to have my mother moved to Ramsey District Cottage Hospital to begin her palliative care, as my father had specifically asked for her to be in Ramsey, for her final days. Dr. Allinson, Judith's G.P. agreed to this. Judith was transferred by ambulance to Ramsey hospital on 22 October, 2012. The day itself was a little bit of a blur. We were all in a constant state of shock and bewilderment.

For Judith the transfer was especially traumatic.

By the time my father, Nigel and myself went in to see Judith, who was still taking I.V. fluid, she was absolutely fuming with anger. She was shouting, swearing and generally abusive. Even her G.P. Dr. Allinson's appearance didn't appease her any.

The irony of the situation was, that here was my mother, literally on death's door after three months of pure hell, and we were apologising for her behaviour to Dr. Allinson.

He was kind enough to take us into an office and explain that Judith was not the person now, that she used to be. He knew how upsetting it was for us, but he told us to focus on our happy times with Judith, and to realise that what we were seeing was not the person that we loved. It was very sweet of him, but the sympathy at such a difficult and horrendous time, made my father very emotional. Empathy often seems to do that under such traumatic circumstances.

Later that night, Sophie went to see her grandmother and took a book to read to her. Judith enjoyed it and listened intently. Sophie explained that she would come the following night to read her some more. Her grandmother said that she would like that.

The following day when we visited, the I.V. fluids had been removed. We had known it would happen, but the reality hit home too hard. My father had brought some food in for Judith, but she refused everything. I managed to get her to take a few sips of water, which she happily accepted. My father himself, looked on death's door too.

We stayed for a few hours, but it was like torture; watching and waiting, knowing that Judith was going to die very soon. I can only imagine the pain of parents watching their children with anorexia refusing to eat. It seems incomprehensible that a person would starve themselves to death. Later that night Sophie went in to read to her grandmother again, which Judith enjoyed yet again. Sophie managed to entice her to take water too.

The next day we saw such a difference in my mother. Her eyes looked sunken, her mouth was crusted, and her hands looked claw-like. She was still talking although the conversation was random and confused. She still had her teddy bear tucked in beside her in bed. Jim brought more food in for Judith, but just the sight of food made her angry. She accepted water though. As she had done on the previous nights, Sophie took the book and read to Judith, who was again, peaceful, calm and listened.

On leaving Sophie explained too, that she would come again the next night to read some more. Judith said, "But I am going to die soon. I don't want to die".

Sophie left the hospital and broke down in tears outside. She rang me explaining this and was so emotional while telling me. We were both sobbing down the phone to each other. Sophie was clearly distraught.

The following day at about 10.00 a.m., the hospital rang to ask us to come straight away to the hospital, as Judith was in her last few hours of life. When Nigel and I arrived, my father was already at Judith's bedside. Judith was in and out of consciousness and her breathing had become laboured. I rang Sophie at work and asked her if she could come to the hospital too. She arrived maybe an hour later.

The nurse asked my father if he wished for a priest or a vicar to be called. Jim hesitated, said, "No", and then five minutes later changed his mind, saying Judith was quite religious and would probably like that. I know that my father was trying to do right by my mother, but the vicar who arrived just seemed annoyingly upbeat, too talkative and his presence I found intrusive. But, on the positive side, it gave my father something to focus on, as they had things in common to talk about. I forget what, but I wished they would just shut-up.

Judith's breathing was becoming shallower, with a rattling noise when she inhaled. We knew that her time was nearing. Sophie and I stood by Judith's bed, one of us either side of her, stroking her hair.

At 14.05 hours, Judith took her last, delicate breath.

The next hour passed in a blur of tears and grief. The vicar said the last rites. The nurse and doctor came in to check the body. The doctor signed the death certificate detailed, "Dementia and essential hypertension". I had watched him write, scrutinising every stroke of the pen – I was curious as to what he would detail.

We individually spent our time with Judith in the ward room. There were mixed emotions of emptiness, sadness, relief and anger. Judith's life had come to a final gruelling end, but my fight for answers as to her demise was just beginning. As I stood, looking over the body of my mother, I instantly realised that day at 4p.m was the meeting at the hospital. I couldn't go. I shouldn't go. It was now inappropriate. Yet, my need for clarity was now even greater. I stared down at my watch. It was 14.45. I could still now make it. The hospital had already attempted to deny me a meeting, perhaps if I cancelled, they might deny it once more.

Despite the trauma and sadness of the moment, I spoke with Sophie and she informed me that she wished to attend the meeting with me. I was most thankful to have her support.

My father was acting unsurprisingly, "not himself". He had pulled the sheet over Judy's face, in a most abrupt and angry manner. He wanted to leave almost immediately. He had phone calls to make and wished to be alone. I tried to insist that he came with us for the evening, but he was insistent on returning home. I decided to follow him to his house to ensure he got in safely and was as comfortable as possible.

From his house, we drove back over the mountain road to our house, in near silence. I had paperwork that I needed to pick up for the meeting too.

Oblivious to the day's events, the dog Kana was overjoyed when we returned. Her excited, beaming doggy smile, reminded me of just how much Judith had loved that little dog. Just that small thought was enough to evoke more tears. After a coffee, and a splash of water on my face, myself and Sophie set off for the meeting. The situation seemed unreal and surreal. The world around me seemed to be operating, without me. I was aware of everything yet felt disassociated from reality. Like somebody watching over events from a birds-eye view.

Sophie and I hugged in the car and walked the frequent path, that we had taken to see my mother, so many times. I could barely walk straight as my legs were shaking, and that tight throat feeling accompanied me, as it had done so often of late.

The person on reception directed us to the meeting room. Upon arrival Amanda Mills was waiting outside of the room for us. In my naivety, I explained that my mother had passed away, just a couple of hours ago, (as if she didn't already know). She stepped forward to embrace me. Just that gesture started my tears again. I attempted to regain my composure quickly. I had to keep strong. I looked at Sophie; she too had tears rolling down her pretty cheeks. We wiped our tears away and headed into the meeting room; my heartbeat inside of me, deafening.

The other members of the meeting were already present – Dr. Tim Byrne, Dr Balakrishnan and Steve Chell, accompanied by Amanda Mills.

Again, I asked to record the meeting. All present agreed to that.

This is a partial transcription of the meeting:-

Dr Byrne, "Would you like to start again for the purpose of the meeting".

Me, "Absolutely. I suspect that my mother suffered neuroleptic malignant syndrome, and this is a direct result of mirtazapine, risperidone and diazepam. I also believe that Dr Jagus and Grianagh Court failed to identify vital signs of this resulting in the undiagnosed state of my mother for over four weeks. A staff member of Ward 5 advised me to make this complaint via this channel. I was going down the route with Dr Jagus and Doreen Fell, but she advised me to go down this road, instead. She went into Ward 1 and 2, and again, I highlighted this swelling. This extreme swelling all around her neck and forearms – they were absolutely solid. I highlighted this again. Just wondering what tests were run in Ward 2?".

Dr Byrne: We wouldn't know. There were blood tests run in Grianagh Court on 20th July".

Me, "At Grianagh Court?"

Dr Byrne, "Yes,".

Me, "I wasn't aware of this".

Dr Byrne, "There was no indication on these blood tests that she was suffering from neuroleptic malignant syndrome. They were being run for different reasons, but they would suggest that she was suffering from an infection. There was a slight increase in white blood cells called neutrophils that would suggest a urinary tract infection. There was concern, from our point of view in Grianagh Court, a suspicion that she might be suffering from an infection that had gone to her kidneys – pyelonephritis and that was the main reason she was referred".

Me, "Days before this, two or three days, she was comatose – she was over sedated. We went in there and she was slumped sideways. She couldn't eat or drink or put a glass to her mouth – she couldn't stand – she couldn't talk. She was completely mute and incapacitated. That went on for three days".

Dr Byrne, "When was this?"

Me, "Probably two or three days prior to when she was admitted to hospital. We raised our concerns about her becoming dehydrated – we couldn't even get a glass to her mouth. Her balance had completely gone. She couldn't even sit up straight, at all. The swelling started in her face and forearms. On 30 May, literally, I remember because it was my birthday, my mother was not wearing Tena lady pants on this occasion; she normally was, she wet herself. I took her to her room to change her and I noticed her calf muscles looked so enlarged, for want of a better word, they looked like footballer's legs. At the time I put it down to her going up and down the corridor constantly. It was such a bizarre looking swelling. I was actually going to ask you to go through her medication on Ward 2, but we don't have that, do we?"

Dr Byrne, "Can I just say just to answer some of the points that you've made – blood tests that were done just before she transferred didn't indicate that she was dehydrated. We ran a test called electrolyte tests. That was on 20th".

Me, "I wasn't aware that tests had been run".

Dr Byrne, "Well I saw them, and they were dated that day".

Me, "I'm not questioning you, I just asked if anything like this had gone on".

Dr Byrne, "The junior doctor that saw her ordered them".

Me, "Prior to my mother being taken into Ward 2 if I can just go through – I spent probably about an hour squeezing water into her mouth from a flannel – squeezing it. Margaret Quayle, (her name is actually Halsall), was there and explained that they used to be able to do this using a sterile gauze, but that this wasn't policy anymore. My mother could not bend her neck; it was as if she was unable to and was shrieking in pain. She appeared to be very thirsty, she had crusted and scabbed lips at the time – her eyes were sunken, and she had dilated pupils. She was sweating and was flushed, and I put another flannel on her forehead to cool her down. Her skin was really strange looking – the only thing I can compare it to, was somebody that I've seen in the chapel of rest, like a very white cold looking skin. Prior to that she was digging her nails into my hand and drew blood, which she has not done before. I thought that she was getting her fight back, but I think she was in a state of heightened agitation and aggression. And again, with neuroleptic malignant syndrome, I would have thought that primary care workers would have noticed the swelling around the neck more than anything".

Dr Byrne, "How would you link that to neuroleptic malignant syndrome?"

Me, "I don't know, I presumed that this was the muscle rigidity, but I've never seen a case of it, so I have no idea".

Dr Byrne, "If there was muscle rigidity it would be unlikely that it would be just limited to the neck".

Me, "Sure, sure, but she had it in her forearms, but I didn't see any other part of her body, so I don't know".

Dr Byrne, "It would be generalised rigidity".

Me, "so this might be through infection then? All this swelling. This swelling was still there when she was sent to Ward 5 though".

Dr Byrne, "I can't comment on it – there is nothing in our records".

Me, "I am hoping that you can see where my concerns are with this amount of swelling".

Dr Byrne, "There was obviously something going on. Her risperidone had been discontinued on 20th because she was drowsy, but she was only on 0.5mg twice a day".

Me, "Her risperidone was actually taken away on 20th (July), completely?"

Dr Byrne, "Completely". (This proved to be untrue. It had been increased to 1mg twice a day, and was then reduced to 0.5mg again, when Judith became unsteady on her feet, along with developing a noticeable tremor).

Me, "Maybe it is a withdrawal symptom then?"

Dr Byrne, "It's very unlikely".

Me, "Very unlikely? Can I just ask, when she was in Ward 5, the nurse said that she was very concerned about the length of time that she had been on risperidone and then asked me if she was on it in Beaconsfield and this is the first time that I knew the drug that she was taking".

Dr Byrne, "Can you remind me of when she was in Beaconsfield?"

Me, "She was in Beaconsfield from.....I forget the date, but she was there up to 2 April".

Dr Byrne, "Right, and she left after that?"

Me, "Yes, she went into Grianagh Court".

Dr Byrne, "Ok again because we don't have records from that time actually, going back, it looks like from what I can see from the records and from what Dr Jagus could see from the records the risperidone was first used on 02 April 2012 so that was after she left. It was stopped on 18 June". (For the record, the duration here is nearly eleven weeks......risperidone in licensed for use in Dementia patients for six weeks only).

Me, "Right, these are all the questions..".

Dr Byrne, "But I can't definitely say that someone didn't prescribe it before".

Me, "Sure, the problem is that, I have here, as well, is that my mother's nurse Delia, when my mother went into a coma-like state, my main highlight was this swelling. I was really concerned about it. It looked like an adverse reaction to something. I asked Delia twice, for a meeting with Dr Jagus, before my mum was admitted to hospital. I then asked her again, no, sorry, she actually rang me at home".

Dr Byrne, "Can I ask you where Delia was? Where was she based?"

Me, "In Grianagh Court".

Steve Chell, "Do you happen to know her surname?"

Me, "I'm afraid, no, sorry I don't"

Dr Byrne, "She must have been based on Elderly",

Me, "I think that she was my mother's named nurse, I think. Sorry, I forget what her surname was".

Dr Byrne, "That's Ok, we can check that".

Steve Chell, "Sorry for interrupting. My limited awareness of the case, I'm sorry but Dr Jagus I believe was willing to meet".

Me, "I think it would be helpful to look at e-mails – there must be some kind of e-mail correspondence, because Delia did say to me at one point that she always e-mailed Dr Jagus. I'm sure she said on a Sunday night. That may be able to locate where the problem lies. I don't know, but I do feel if we'd have been able to have this meeting, I could have asked a lot more questions at that point. Also, from Grianagh Court aspect, when my mother was in Ward 2 and we were still waiting for this meeting to go on, a clear bin bag with my mother's clothing got dumped into the room which I thought seemed very disrespectful. Somebody could have rang and asked us to come and collect the belongings and we could have folded them up and put them in a case, rather than just literally thrown into a clear bin bag and put in the room, but that's only a minor issue".

Steve Chell, "I apologise for that".

Me, "That's only a minor issue, so, sorry. In the meeting on 07 September, that we had, Dr Jagus stated that my mother's coma-like state prevented her from taking medication that he had prescribed and seemed to think that therefore he didn't need to withdraw the drugs in question. Is this true that she didn't take any more risperidone or Mirtazapine or Diazepam since she was in hospital?"

Dr Byrne, "As far as I can see – again, I would have to check. She didn't get any more risperidone".

Me, "She didn't the whole time she was in Noble's?"

Dr Byrne, "As far as I can see it was withdrawn".

Dr Balakrishnan, "Unfortunately, I was away on the twenty fifth. I think she was admitted the day that I went on annual leave and I was back on sixth. I was told about her condition and I think you had a meeting with Dr Jagus on Ward 5 on 08 September".

Me, "We did yes. I think I put it in my letter as 07 September".

Dr Balakrishnan, "I think I met you the following week".

Me, "Yes. So, she didn't take any risperidone the whole time she was in Noble's?"

Dr Balakrishnan, "I can't inform without seeing the notes".

Amanda Mills, "We'll get these from Ramsey".

Me, "I actually wondered if they had been given to her in liquid form. That's confusing, actually with what the sister was telling me on Ward 5, Michelle, she actually brought up the risperidone with me. I don't understand why she would have brought that up with me, or why that was mentioned. I really don't understand that at all otherwise".

Dr Byrne, "We don't understand that either".

Me, "No, I really don't understand that".

Amanda Mills, "What did Michelle ask you?"

Me," She said that they were concerned about the length of time that she's been on risperidone".

Dr Byrne, "I wonder whether she was a little confused at the time".

Me, "She also seemed to be under the impression that she was still at Beaconsfield".

Dr Byrne, "Ok but even that was in April, as far as we know and I have to say that I don't know what happened at Beaconsfield, but she wasn't on it when she came to Grianagh Court".

Me, "She wasn't?"

Dr Byrne, "It was commenced then, stopped in June and restarted on 14 July and stopped on 20 July".

Me, "Right".

Dr Byrne, "There is nothing that would suggest a long time, and she was on a small dose".

Me, "Obviously, up to this point I was not aware of the drugs that my mother was on. As another side of it, I believe that it would have been nice if we'd been called in to a meeting and told of the drugs she was on and of the high risks involved with risperidone".

Dr Byrne, "Can I stop you there. Can you tell me who told you there were high risks?"

Me, "This is from what I have been reading and from the Alzheimer's Society especially".

Dr Byrne, "Did they give you any indication of what the level, or how often this happens".

Me, "How often?"

Dr Byrne, "Somebody might develop neuroleptic malignant syndrome?"

Me, "They couldn't on that, no".

Dr Byrne, "OK".

Me, "That wasn't what they....".

Dr Byrne, "Ok it would be helpful if I gave you an idea".

Me, "I believe that it is very few and far between".

Dr Byrne, "Risperidone is one of the least likely drugs to cause it".

Me, "It's one of the atypical ones, yes, but it is very much linked to it. I know it's a very rare condition. I am aware of that yes. How many have been detected on the island?".

Dr Byrne, "Well, I can't remember. I'm sure there probably have been some on the island. I can't remember one in my experience over the last number of years. It happens in less than one per cent of people who ever receive antipsychotic or neuroleptic drugs".

Me, "That's reported".

Dr Byrne, "That's reported – it is much less likely to happen on the newer drugs such as risperidone and it's much less likely to happen when people get it in small amounts, as your mum did".

Me, "I have actually gone through Medlink Neurology and various different places and actually bought reports on neuroleptic malignant syndrome. It is directly linked to risperidone. It is one of the prolific atypical antipsychotics".

Dr Byrne, "It is one of the ones that is used often – yes".

Me, "For dementia, absolutely".

Dr Byrne, "It's the only one that's licensed for it".

Me, "Yes I am aware of that. Do we operate a yellow card scheme over here?"

Dr Byrne, "Yes".

Me, "We do. Then we will know how many cases of neuroleptic malignant syndrome have been on the island and specifically at Grianagh Court as well, perhaps".

Dr Byrne, "We could find out perhaps, it depends, the information would be kept in a database in the UK. We could find out?"

Steve Chell, "We could endeavour to do so".

Me, "Yes, that would be great. I'd be very interested to see that".

Dr Byrne, "You're talking about somewhere under one per cent. It is probable that somebody developed it here over the years, but again, I think we must put this into context. It is usually people who are on much higher levels of these medications".

Me, "Not necessarily higher levels, I have done research and have got some back up here".

Dr Byrne, "I am not saying always, I'm saying it is possible".

Me, "But on this side of it there are certain aspects of it, my mother's condition that cannot be explained medically".

Dr Byrne, "Can you tell me what particular pieces would suggest neuroleptic malignant syndrome. It wasn't suggested to anyone else. That's my difficulty".

Me, "I did ask Dr Bajeed (actually Majeed), if I could just run through this. Ok, excuse me for reading it. I explained my own concerns to Dr Bajeed when I was visiting my mother in Ward 5, after explaining how she was overly-sedated in Grianagh Court, following an increase in medication and asked if she might have neuroleptic malignant syndrome. He explained that they were going to run some tests and scans. A few days later he explained that the CT and MRI scans were clear, as was the lumbar puncture, and at this point Dr Bajeed did not tell me how difficult the lumbar puncture was. He did mention that it was clear and he said that it looked like my suspicions were right and that the dementia drugs were going to be withdrawn and that we should see an improvement in her condition over the next four days or so, which we did and it was blatantly clear. We did see an improvement in her condition after that".

Dr Byrne, "The difficulty is she didn't appear, unless she was put back on those drugs when she was admitted. She wasn't admitted on them. They were stopped".

Me, "She might well have been, but the fact that she was put on them for a few days and then stopped. That could actually induce Neuroleptic Malignant Syndrome too".

Dr Byrne, "Again, it's very unlikely. She was on the tiniest amount".

Me, "It might be unlikely, but it is possible".

Dr Byrne, "Ok, I am suggesting that it is possible, but what I am asking you is what were the indications that she was. You've told me nothing yet that suggests that she was suffering from it".

Me, "She had a high temperature when she was admitted".

Dr Byrne, "That's not necessarily, the temperature actually fluctuates. How high was her temperature? The temperature reading, the highest temperature reading at Grianagh Court was 38.5 – that's not a particularly high temperature".

Me, "OK can I just ask, key points. Neuroleptic malignant syndrome is a life-threatening condition and should be suspected in anyone taking a dopamine receptor blocking drug, who has a high fever, or a decline in the level of alertness. That's all three".

Dr Byrne, "OK".

Me, "OK. A diagnosis of neuroleptic malignant syndrome is clinical and may be impossible to distinguish from coincident infection; both may be present. OK?"

Dr Byrne, "OK".

Me, "Although there is a disagreement about treatment options, all would agree that the offending drug must be stopped".

Dr Byrne, "But I am saying to you, there are lots and lots of conditions that could involve a high temperature".

Me, "Sure, sure".

Dr Byrne, "And people would take these things into account, there are lots of other symptoms that would need to be present to give us some reason to suspect......".

Me, "I think maybe because it is called neuroleptic malignant syndrome – malignant being the main word here and my mother is actually dead. Evidence. Not evidence of that, but evidence of something more serious, that all these tests showed were clear, was actually there".

Dr Byrne, "I realise that you are upset, and I am sorry for that and I'm really sorry that we're having this conversation at this time. Could you please explain to me what you mean by what you said? You said the word, "Malignant". that implies in some way, that this caused your mother's death".

Me, "Yes, that's exactly what I am saying – that it is a life threatening condition and it's also linked with catatonia, which can include a refusal to eat, and as Dr Krishnan here knows, my Mum has not eaten for twelve weeks and she point blank refused. She had anorexia, which is one of the symptoms of neuroleptic malignant syndrome in general, if you can explain it in any other way, please do."

Dr Byrne, "Sure, can I please explain what the word, "Malignant", is and refers to. It refers to a very quickly changing set of symptoms and signs that change quickly, it's nothing to do with cancer or anything like that".

Me, "Yes, I am aware of that. Yes".

Dr Byrne. I, I, I really don't want to appear patronising, but it's important that we're clear about what we are saying".

Me, "Absolutely".

Dr Byrne, "Just going back, the difficulty with any medical diagnosis is there are lots and lots of possibilities".

Me, "I appreciate that".

Dr Byrne, "We have to consider various possibilities. We have to look at what is most likely and we have to investigate by investigations. We do that by examining the patient physically and observing the patient and by running various laboratory tests. Now these things were done and done appropriately and none of the things that the doctors could see or the results of the tests suggested that she had neuroleptic malignant syndrome. The only suspicion seems to be coming from the Dr., I've forgotten his name, does it begin with a "B"?"

Dr Balakrishnan, "Majeed, but he didn't say that, I think he said that it may be a possibility".

Me, "But the fact was that he was going to withdraw the drugs and in four days or so, we should see an improvement. That was fact. We did see an improvement. She actually had to be moved into a side-ward eventually, because she was talking too much. Previous to that she was mute. She was hardly talking at all".

Dr Byrne, "She was being treated for a Urinary Tract infection and a very large gallstone".

Me, "She's had that previously, yes".

Dr Byrne, "The most common reason for sedation, confusion and perhaps refusal to eat would be physical problems, the infection and she would have been treated with antibiotics".

Me, "Sure, which didn't make any improvement in her mental status".

Dr Byrne, "Usually it takes a little bit longer for the mental state to improve, until the infection improves. What you are saying fits very much into the infection".

Me, "But what about the periods of time, when she didn't have an infection? Nobody knew what was wrong with her. There didn't appear to be any infection present".

Dr Byrne, "But there was infection before".

Me, "But surely if you left her with neuroleptic malignant syndrome and that wasn't treated, surely she would develop and get another infection?"

Dr Byrne, "There's no connection between the two".

Me, "Ok let me just go onto the next bit, in that case. Without my mother's notes actually being here, which is what I was led to believe would happen, I can't actually ask a lot more questions, that I wanted to. There seemed to be quite a sustained period in Ward 5 where nobody could explain what was wrong with her".

Dr Balakrishnan, "Will have to check the case notes and see".

Me, "Later the diagnosis of Cholecystitis was made and treated. We didn't see any improvement in her mental alertness then, and then again there seemed to be a period of uncertainty again. Dr Majeed informed us that my mother was given fourteen days of antibiotics for suspected Encephalitis.

Dr Krishnan, "That was a clinical diagnosis. She was not getting better and because of the confusion. She was suspected of viral Encephalitis, for the herpes simplex and giving her antiviral treatment, but it didn't make any difference".

Me, "No, it didn't make any difference at all, no. I was just going to ask, what were the suspicions for the Encephalitis but they were clinical. There weren't any tests done to prove that at all".

Dr Krishnan, "But she had the lumbar puncture and that didn't suggest a viral infection".

Me, "Yes, those were all clear".

Steve Chell, "Sorry, may I interrupt again. You made reference to medications being stopped and then there was a noticeable improvement. What medication?"

Me, "Again, that's what I was going to ask with my mother's notes".

Dr Balakrishnan, "We need to see the notes".

Me, "Again, Ward 1 and 2 stated that they were concerned about her medication, that appeared to be making her drowsy. She was just sleeping and couldn't eat or drink. I was going to ask if that was in her case notes as well.

Dr Byrne, "When she went over to Noble's hospital she wasn't getting any medication".

Me, "Right".

Dr Byrne, "I can't say what happened when she came over, but that had all been stopped". (untrue – all medication had carried on, despite a psychiatric meds review on 21 July; just one day after her medical ward admission).

Me, "It had? Definitely? That's where I am puzzled".

Dr Balakrishnan, "I can't answer that without the notes".

Me, "I am puzzled as to why I would have been told that in hospital too, that we would see this improvement in four days' time".

Dr Balakrishnan, "We need to see the notes".

Amanda Mills, "We will get them".

Me, "Definitely, and after that period why, coincidentally, we did see an improvement, this drastic improvement in her alertness and talking, along with being able to respond to people".

Dr Balakrishan, "What period are we talking – end of August?"

Me, "Yes, I think it was around the end of August, yes. I am sure it was around 26 August, somewhere like that".

Dr Krishnan, "We will need to see the case notes, because I came back to work on 06 September. She was still completely unconscious, not co-operative. By this time, they had done all the investigations and all the test and bloods were fine. CT/MRI and lumbar puncture were all fine. All the possible medical conditions considered and treated, but no explanation to her condition".

The meeting went on to further discussions about dehydration :-

Me, "I think the fact that you can't hold a drink or hold a cup, and even if someone puts it to your mouth, is a clear factor that somebody is likely to become dehydrated, on this medication that she shouldn't be allowed to dehydrate on".

Dr Byrne, "We were attempting to admit her".

Me, "I know, but I get the feeling that if my father and me weren't actually visiting her, it would have been delayed a lot longer. It was only the fact that we were jumping up and down stamping our feet a little bit, that she got in earlier, in all honesty and in fairness to all of you".

Dr Byrne, "Can I just ask you, who do you think was blocking the admission?"

Me, "I don't think anyone was blocking the admission necessarily,

I think people were not as concerned as we were. I think that is probably fair enough to say. Just going through the facts here. Dr Jagus in the meeting in Ward 5 said that neuroleptic malignant syndrome was a possibility. I have that on the recording of the last meeting. If that was the case and he thought it was a possibility, then I think he should have....I mean I believe that the drugs were stopped now from what you are telling me, but I asked him and he said he didn't feel any need to withdraw them because she was so drowsy".

The meeting continued to discuss other issues, but without my mother's medical notes, nothing could be clarified.

Lots of times, Amanda Mills informed me that would be get my mother's notes. It took some months and a formal application before I had access to them. At one point Judith's medical notes were "lost".

I had asked also for the risperidone patient information leaflet to be present at the meeting, requested on 18 October. This was never produced at the meeting either.

Outside the meeting, Sophie and I both agreed what an arrogant, condescending man Dr Byrne was. I didn't trust him and with good reason, it would prove. Little did I know, but he was a Psychiatrist too.

Dr Byrne has since been removed from the Doctors' Register by the GMC. He was having a relationship with his vulnerable patient for two years. This period covered the dates that Judith was in the unit and the hospital.

21

Funeral Arrangements

The next week was a scurry of activity, as in every case when a loved one dies. Engaging the funeral service; writing the obituary; registering the death; informing family and friends; arranging funeral service. The list was endless. To make matters worse, my father appeared to be in meltdown, and denial, coupled with anger, along with no sense of reality. I was very concerned for his mental health, and his high risk of another stroke. My father wanted almost nothing to do with the funeral arrangements.

I went with the undertaker, to register my mother's death at the Registrar's Office in Douglas. I parked my car outside of the offices and met him on the forecourt. We were filling in the form quite straight forwardly, until I came to a part that asked if there was a negligence case involved with the deceased. I hesitated, then told the undertaker that there was. He then explained that if I declared this, then the funeral would be postponed, following a possible enquiry, and that this could take some considerable time. I thought briefly, and decided that following the meeting and being told that my mother's medication had been stopped upon her admission to hospital, which was the most crucial point that I was trying to relay, that maybe there was little point in causing further disruption, and more importantly, unnecessary further stress to my father. The undertaker informed me that I would also need to cancel the flights that I had just booked for all the family members, if I declared the negligence issue. With all of this in mind, in a few split seconds I made the decision to refrain from informing the office that there was a negligence case regarding Judith's death. I was aware of the penalty for doing this but decided to proceed with non-declaration. We sat in the Registrar's office, while a librarian-type looking gentleman completed the official register. When it came to the Cause of Death he stopped and explained that "Dementia", was not a valid reason for death. The registrar's assistant explained that he needed to speak with the doctor who had signed the death certificate, before the registering of Judith's death could be completed.

The undertaker and me sat in the waiting room. He paced a little, looking at his watch, becoming distinctly anxious. He then sat down next to me and informed me that this could take a long time, waiting for the doctor to become available to speak with the Registrar officer. The undertaker explained the he had a very busy schedule and week ahead. His sense of self-importance annoyed me.

Luckily, only ten or fifteen minutes passed before the Registrar's assistant informed us that he had spoken with the doctor and that would enable us to finalise the registering of the death. I felt very uneasy with the process, and in hindsight needed more time to ponder the issue of negligence. I have come to realise that I made an error of judgement on this. The findings of any autopsy could have been immensely useful in discovering more, with regards to neuroleptic malignant syndrome, and possible, Lewy Bodies Dementia. Yet, with the protecting climate surrounding the Isle of Man NHS, I suspect that there was a sizeable chance that this would not have happened too.

The following day, I received a letter from Amanda Mills at the hospital, detailing that she would be in a position to review my mother's medical notes during the week commencing 05 November 2012. I guessed that would take some considerable time.

Running up to the funeral was very busy with arrangements and with members of Judith's family coming over to the island; most were staying at our house, and one member I had arranged a hotel for two nights, as sleeping arrangements necessitated. Our house would be full-to-capacity, which in all honesty, I was dreading. I desperately need alone time, but this was not going to happen anytime soon.

Evening times I was undertaking further research on risperidone and neuroleptic malignant syndrome. I had no previous idea of the controversy surrounding the two, let alone the connection between them. I now learned that risperidone was the only antipsychotic medication licensed for use in elderly people with dementia, for the treatment of dementia-related behavioural disturbances, as Dr Byrne had told me, and that it was only licensed for short-term use, (up to six weeks) Treatment of persistent aggression in Alzheimer's dementia, unresponsive to non-pharmacological approaches, and where there was a risk of harm to the patient and others. I knew that my mother had been prescribed risperidone for longer than the short-term six weeks, in fact eleven weeks, as Dr Byrne informed me in the meeting.

The Medicines and Healthcare Products Agency; a U.K Government Agency, (MHRA), detailed that elderly people with dementia are at a risk from specific serious and life-threatening side-effects, when treated with antipsychotics. Risperidone, (Risperdal), was a, "black triangle" status drug, when used in the elderly dementia population. This means that medicine with this category is subject to intensive monitoring. Suspected adverse reactions can be reported online at www.yellowcard.mhra.gov.uk. For risperidone, there was an additional increase in the risk of mortality when co-prescribed with furosemide; a diuretic. (ref: Drug Safety Update, March 2009. Vol 1 issue 8:5).

MHRA, "Drug Safety Update", latest advice for medicine users, detailed:-

"There have been increasing concerns over recent years about the use of antipsychotic to treat behavioural and psychological symptoms in dementia, (BPSD). Antipsychotics are associated with an increased risk of cerebrovascular adverse events, and a greater mortality.

<u>National Dementia Strategy for England.</u>

In 2009, in the face of identified shortcomings in the provision of dementia services in the UK and with the increasing challenge to society posed by dementia, the government announced the first National Dementia Strategy for England.

The Government commissioned the Banerjee Report, ("Time for Action"; an independent review of the use of antipsychotic in elderly dementia patients). The report concluded that antipsychotic use was too high in patients with dementia, and the associated risks outweighed the benefit in most of these patients."

Another article that I stumbled across was an article by Ewan Maule, (in the British Journal of Clinical Pharmacy. July/August 2009. Vol. 1). Ewan Maule was a clinical pharmacist for emergency and critical care at Northumbria Healthcare NHS Foundation Trust, at the time:-

Management of Neuroleptic Malignant Syndrome.

Neuroleptic malignant syndrome (NMS), is a rare but potentially fatal neurological complication of treatment with antipsychotic drugs, (historically called neuroleptics). It can also develop upon withdrawal of some anti-parkinsonian medications, although this is rare. NMS is an idiopathic condition that occurs in some patients, although its mechanism is not fully understood.

About 80% of cases of NMS develop within the first two weeks of antipsychotic use, but can occur at any point during therapy. Risperidone is one of the drugs associated with NMS, amongst others.

Clinical Symptoms of NMS.

Altered mental status: drowsiness, progressing to stupor and coma.

Pyrexia: temperature typically 38 degrees Celsius and above.

Autonomic dysfunction: usually tachycardia or labile blood pressure.

Muscle rigidity: often described as, "lead pipe rigidity".

Tachypnea, (rapid breathing).

Diaphoresis, (Excessive sweating).

Drooling.

Incontinence.

Biochemical Symptoms.
Raised creatine kinase, usually in excess of 1,000 IU/L. Levels up to 100,000 IU/L have been reported.

Leukocytosis; present in up to 75% of cases.

Iron deficiency.

Liver function abnormalities.

Treatment and Management.
The most important and effective treatment of NMS is cessation of the causative drug and any other implicated psychotropic medication, followed by supportive care.

The recovery time after cessation of the causative drug is usually seven to 10 days. However, this may be longer if the causative drug was administered by a depot injection: **rare cases of residual catatonia and motor signs have been reported up to six months after cessation of causative drug.**

There is no "gold standard", treatment for NMS and drug use is largely unsupported by evidence. However, pharmacological interventions are frequently used because of the relatively high rates of morbidity and mortality in patients with NMS.

Electroconvulsive Therapy.
If pharmacological agents are ineffective despite adequate dosing, then ECT can be considered. The evidence supporting ECT is not easily comparable because of the wide variation in how and when it is used with respect to the onset of NMS. However, a study has shown lower mortality rate in ECT-treated patients compared with those receiving supportive care, (10.3% and 21% respectively).

Conclusions.
Pharmacists can play an important role in the management of NMS by recognizing symptoms, identifying causative medication, establishing a treatment plan and reporting outcomes.

As our understanding of NMS and its treatment improves, and as newer antipsychotics are developed, the incidences of NMS should reduce and survival rates improve.

(Please see above reference link for the full article).

Other articles (Medscape. Neuroleptic Malignant Syndrome Clinical presentation. Author J Tonkonogy et al), detailed the clinical features of NMS to be:-

Diaphoresis
Dysphagia
Tremor
Incontinence
Delirium progressing to lethargy, stupor and coma.
Labile blood pressure.
Pallor
Dyspnea.
Psychomotor agitation.
Rigidity.
Hyperthermia.
Tachycardia.
Shuffling gait.

Without my mother's medical notes, I seemed at a loss to cite all or most of these symptoms.

22
The Funeral

A couple of days before my mother's funeral, my family members arrived. Bryan Judith's brother and his wife Cherie, and their beautiful daughter; my cousin, Jeanette, and Judith's sister Ruth. It was lovely to see them, but I suspect that I was suffering from depression. I really had to try hard to appear happy or enthusiastic about anything. I just wished that I could snap out of it. I felt as if I was in a constant state of shock and not in the "real world". I was feeling no pleasure in anything; not even the beauty of the surrounding trees and bird song that I normally appreciated so much. Kana, the dog, raised my spirits a little, but even her barking, which I normally found amusing, was irritating me. Every morning, just getting out of bed was an effort. Showering made me think about death. Nigel's presence I found annoying. I truly felt that I was going crazy. I wanted to get-away from myself. I hated myself. I dreaded to think how my father was coping. I put a brave face on and settled everybody into their rooms. My cousin was sleeping in the lounge on a recently sourced camp bed. I hoped that she would be comfortable and warm enough.

I had made arrangements for my mother to be visited at the chapel of rest. The undertaker was to ring me the previous day to inform me of a suitable time to visit, but I had not heard from him. I decided to ring him instead. His wife answered, and curtly explained that he was very busy and it might not be possible; that he had not said that he would ring me. I begged to differ with her and explained that I had family members over and informed her that this was the service that we were paying for. The fact that he was busy was effectively, not our problem, and I asked her to get him to ring me back. I came off the phone, shocked by her attitude.

Some ten minutes later, he called back and explained that we could come and visit in half an hour, if that suited us. I accepted the allotted time and thanked him.

Half an hour later, we were outside the funeral home. Sophie met us there too. It was a cold day but stepping in through the chapel of rest front door was even colder and damper. The smell was musty. Bryan did not wish to see his sister now; he wished to remember her, as he had last seen her, on 23 March 2012 on Jim and Judy's anniversary.

The undertaker took us in to see my mother. She looked peaceful. That was the first thing that I noticed, having seen her in such anguish and pain for those last three months.

Sophie had asked previously, for the funeral director to colour Judith's hair roots, as my daughter commented that her grandmother's hair had always been immaculate with never a grey hair in sight. It had seemed an unusual request, but it made my mother look like her old self.

We then all came back out and went in individually to say our goodbyes. I went inside to see my mother for the last time. I apologised to her for everything that she had been through and vowed to fight the cause. In a split second I retreated back. I half expected my mother to jump up and start shouting at me. The mind plays tricks when under such sadness and stress. The tears started rolling. Tears of both sadness and guilt. My anxiety kicked in, and I rushed out for fresh air.

We all got back into the cars and returned to our house. Everybody talked about how much weight Judy had lost, and how she didn't look like Judy anymore. Bryan was quiet. He had terminal cancer, and the whole thing must have been quite traumatic for him.

Once back at the house, I went quickly into the bedroom, then into the en-suite and vomited. I felt sick to the pit of my stomach.

My mother's cousin, Gordon, was to arrive the night before the funeral and was staying in a hotel for a couple of nights. That night prior to the funeral we met Gordon down at the Sefton Hotel on Douglas seafront. The drinks were flowing, and Gordon ordered bottle after bottle of red wine. We all sat around chatting about good times and remembering Judith.

I felt tortured just listening. I had come to the conclusion that I had failed my mother so desperately. Perhaps if I had focused more on my research, then I could have helped her sooner; been braver and demanded answers; been bolder and questioned relentlessly; not been so meek in my approach; not been intimidated by my lack of knowledge. I was utterly disgusted with myself. I could barely live with knowing that I had not protected my mother from such an adverse reaction to medication. I indulged in more and more red wine. It numbed my sense of guilt and utter revulsion about myself. My sense of pleasure and humour heightened as the alcohol soothed me and took hold. My relationship with the intoxication was rekindled after a period of abstinence. I had arrived into the Sefton, Norman Wisdom's bar looking near immaculate, but I was now leaving as a total wreck; legs barely able to move on my tottering high heeled boots.

Gordon had departed, leaving us waiting at the taxi rank outside. I could only just stand, so sat accompanying the life-size bronze statue of Norman Wisdom sitting on a bench. I took the space on the bench beside him, put my arms around him, then promptly bathed him in a warm flow of red wine vomit. Moments later a taxi arrived. My family piled into the back of the taxi. The taxi driver refused to take me. Nigel gave my relatives the door key to let themselves in and remained with me, understandably angry and disgusted.

Sometime later, the Polish taxi driver returned and relented on taking me home. I was so thankful to him. Such a kind soul. My family had pleaded my case on their way home.

Waking up the next morning for me, was like raising the dead. Very apt on the day of my mother's funeral. Thankfully, the funeral cars were picking my father up from Ramsey and then the two cars would come to our house. My horrendous hangover kept me from beating myself up. My focus was on not vomiting again.

My father, myself, Nigel, Sophie and her partner, Chris went in one car. The remaining family members followed in the second car. There was near silence in the car until Nigel picked up conversation with Sophie and Chris. My father looked so frail and grey. His bottom lip was quivering. I so desperately wanted to hug him, but I just squeezed the back of his neck, from the rear of the car.

When we arrived at the crematorium Jim got out of the car and I went around to hold him, but his legs just buckled. Luckily Nigel was on the opposite side of me, so we held him up between us, supporting him as we walked in. The vicar who had been at my mother's bedside at her point of death, was taking the service. Still I didn't warm to him any. He knew our feelings on Judith's demise with the Mental Health service and briefly touched on our concerns. The service for me was somewhat of a blur. My heart was banging and my throat was again taut with anxiety.

After the service, we waited patiently as everybody came out of the crematorium. I was utterly disgusted to see Marie and Diane from the Mental Health Service line up to offer their condolences. Just for that day, I wished to forget about the Mental Health Services. I saw the look on their faces when they saw me. My complaint had obviously riled them. In my opinion they were not welcome, but I ensured that after hugging my father, they had to embrace me too. It was a half-hearted forced embrace. I wanted to ask them if they had come to ensure the cremation was final. Couldn't they leave us in peace, even now? I calmed myself down. Was I being, "spectrum special", again?

We had invited everybody back to the Creg-ny-Baa Restaurant and bar. A place that Judith had loved going as a family. We had for the past few years been there on Boxing Day. Some very special times had been had. It seemed especially suitable for the Wake. My father had refused to have a free bar – he didn't want people enjoying Judith's demise, so coffee, tea and a wonderful buffet spread was put on.

Normally a time for the celebration of a person's life, we felt a burden of guilt and injustice.

I made my excuses for a short time to go and let Kana out, but I needed to go home for at least ten minutes alone. I was overwhelmed and desperately in need of vomiting.

I returned after maybe fifteen minutes. Hopefully nobody had noticed that I had left. Nigel had told me it was totally unacceptable, but I didn't care. I slipped back into the Creg-ny-Baa, picked up a plate and tried to eat some food, and attempted small talk with whoever wished. My father was holding up well, considering how ill he looked. After most people had left, he insisted that I order him a taxi back to Ramsey. He didn't want to come back to my house. I wanted to be with my father, but I had a house full of family to attend to.

Back at our house, the drinks flowed some more and I later prepared some food.

I really wasn't in the mood for any kind of social gathering. Nigel appeared to be enjoying the red wine and was deep in conversation. I took the opportunity to make my excuses and headed off to bed, thankful for the quietness and alone time. I just sobbed and was relieved that nobody could see me.

23
The Aftermath

On 15th November, I received a letter from Amanda Mills, detailing that the investigation into my complaint and the points raised, was still ongoing.

I carried on relentlessly with my research into NMS. What I discovered really alarmed me. This rare illness was in fact profoundly known about. The Alzheimer's Society were quite prolific in the campaign against antipsychotic overuse in the elderly dementia population; it being prescribed off-licence, and the inappropriate use of the medication too.

I wrote an e-mail to the Alzheimer's helpline and explained the course of events with my mother, to them.

Part of the Alzheimer's Society response was :-

"In your mother's case it sounds as though she may have developed NMS as a result of being prescribed with three types of neuroleptics at once. Although I can't comment on how often this occurs, I'm shocked to hear that this has happened. I would suggest that you consider making a formal complaint to the NHS against the action of prescribing this medication against licence, but also in combination with other similar antipsychotic medication". He went on to offer advice on the pathways to take, in order to do this.

The Isle of Man has different procedures, its own Government and laws, and is in fact, "protected", from the UK complaints route. I have my suspicions that the fact of this, makes the Isle of Man NHS very complacent and is resulting in not learning from its own mistakes, or rather, not admitting to its own mistakes in the first place.

I received a letter from the Isle of Man Hospital dated 11 December 2012 :-

"Dear Mrs Quine
Thank you for your letter dated 04 October 2012 which we received on 05 October 2012. May we firstly offer our sincere condolences on the sad loss of your mother and we are sorry that you have had cause to complain at this sad time. We have investigated your concerns with the help of the Mental Health Service and Surgical Divisions at Noble's Hospital under Local Resolution of the Isle of Man NHS Complaints Procedure. We are also aware that you met with staff members from the Mental Health Service and from Noble's Hospital on 25 October to discuss your concerns. This meeting was recorded at your request and with the permission of those present: Mr Steve Chell, Head of Mental Health Services; Dr Tim Byrne, Consultant Psychiatrist and Clinical Director, Mental Health Services; Dr Balakrishnan, Consultant Physician and Amanda Mills, Case Manager.

Please accept our apologies for the delay in providing you with this response. This has been due to the fact that different areas were involved in your mother's care and we wanted to ensure that you received as comprehensive a reply as possible.

We felt it would be helpful if we firstly gave an overview of your mother's care and then commented specifically on the concerns that you have raised in your letter.

As you are aware your mother was first referred to Dr Jagus in the latter part of 2008. She had a diagnosis of Alzheimer's disease of relatively early onset; her being in her mid-sixties when she started with it. Dr Jagus has noted that you mother's dementia was characterised throughout with very high levels of depression, distress, irritability and aggression. Indeed, when she was first referred it was difficult to assess her cognitive function because of the presence of significant depressive symptoms which were being treated at the time with Mirtazapine. Mirtazapine has been used throughout the course of her unfortunate and rapidly-progressing illness, as many depressive features continued throughout the illness. In the early stages of her illness a diagnosis was by no means clear and it was only during 2010 that it became clear that what she was suffering from was dementia. At this point she was commenced on Donezepil and she was also taking Memantine as a combination therapy, in an attempt to treat her dementia. Unfortunately, her dementia proved very difficult to treat.

Your mother was ultimately admitted to Grianagh Court on 30 October 2011 after increasing escalating levels of verbal and physical aggression towards both her husband who cared for her and you. Your father sadly suffered a stroke and was admitted to Noble's Hospital.

Your mother was discharged in December 2011 to Glen House Care Home but whilst there, as you are aware, she displayed significant episodes of agitation and aggression towards others. Your mother moved to Beaconsfield Nursing Home in Ramsey at the beginning of February 2012. Sadly, the problems with high levels of distress, tearfulness, agitation and aggression continued at the home and she was finally admitted back to Grianagh Court under Section 2 of the Mental Health Act on 02 April 2012. Her management had remained problematic throughout with little alleviation of her behavioural symptoms, despite appropriate nursing and environmental management. It was felt necessary in the circumstances and because of the high risk to herself and/or others to utilise neuroleptic drugs to try and settle her behaviours. There are also documented reports of psychotic symptoms including hallucinations which would equally make their use appropriate.

Your mother was admitted to Noble's Hospital on 20 July 2012. Leading up to this, there had been continued evidence of agitation and aggression along with some reports of visual hallucinations. Dr Jagus had noted on 12 July 2012 that there was a report of increased urinary frequency and urgency with cloudy urine. With her urine heavily positive for nitrate and leucocytes, (an indication that an infection was present), your mother was prescribed Nitrofurantoin (an antibiotic) 250mgs four times daily, at this point.

It was documented by staff at Grianagh Court that your mother continued to remain agitated and was kicking and biting staff in the days following this. Your mother was reviewed by Dr Marie O'Sullivan on 14 July 2012 and commenced on Risperidone 0.5mg twice a day. However, during the ward round, carried out by Dr Marie O'Sullivan, Locum Consultant (as Dr Jagus was on annual leave at this stage), two days later it was noted that there was continued evidence of disturbed behaviours, visual hallucinations and aggression towards other patients, visitors and staff and her Risperidone was increased at this point.

On 17 July2012, your mother was noted by staff to be slightly less resistive and aggressive and on 18 July noted to be slightly unsteady on her feet and a little drowsy, but still pacing the ward. It is reported that Dr. O'Sullivan reduced her risperidone on 19 July 2012 back to 0.5mgs twice a day. In the evening of 19 July 2012 your mother was observed to be drowsy and unsteady on her feet, walking with a stooped gait and her temperature at this point was 36.6 degrees. On the morning of 20 July 2012, it was noted that she continued to be drowsy, resistive and hostile. She drank a glass of juice at this point but was not chewing her sandwich and staff believed this was due to her continued drowsiness. Her medication was withheld because of concerns about sedation.

Your mother was reviewed by Dr Kjell-Arne Nordgard and in an entry dated 20 July 2012 at 15.16 hours, he noted that your mother was drowsy with newly-developed rashes on her legs. She had a temperature of 37.4 degrees and her blood pressure and heart rate were recorded as within expected limits. She was very somnolent and drowsy. She needed assistance from staff when transferring to bed. She would open her eyes when being examined but was not responding well to staff.

On examination, your mother was noted to have a dry tongue, but no sign of lymphadenopathy (swollen lymph glands) or anaemia. There was no leg swelling but it was noted there was a recently developed papular (raised) rash on her shins. Other examination was normal apart from tenderness in the left loin and therefore Dr Nordgard's differential diagnosis was pyelonephritis, despite her being on Nitrofurantoin. He took bloods and she was referred to Ward 2 Noble's Hospital and at that point her temperature was 38.5, but she was maintaining normal blood pressure.

Your mother was admitted to Ward 1 (as there were no beds on Ward 2, the Female Surgical ward). Staff on the ward recall that your mother was sleepy at times, but assessed that this was due to her being unwell and weak with the infection Your mother was treated with intravenous fluids and antibiotics and on 25 July 2012 she was reviewed by the surgical team who assessed that she was medically fit to return to Grianagh Court. Your mother was transferred back on 27 July 2012.

On her transfer back to Grianagh Court staff noted that your mother remained lethargic and that her temperature was recorded as 37.3 degrees (slightly elevated). There was concern that she was not medically fit and your mother had been transferred back to Noble's Hospital on 28 July 2012 for further assessment and treated if indicated. It was at this point, we have been informed that you raised your first concern that your mother's physical state may be due to her medication.

Your mother was admitted to the Medial Assessment Unit (MAU) at Noble's Hospital at 14.00 hours on 28 July 2012. She was seen and examined by Dr Ibrahim, Foundation Year

1 Doctor at 16.00 hours and initial investigations were carried out and a treatment plan drawn up. Your mother was reviewed by Dr Khuraijam, Locum Consultant Physician at 17.20 hour, on his ward round where a diagnosis of cholecystitis (inflammation of the gall bladder) due to gall stones was made. Intravenous fluids and antibiotics were commenced.

Your mother was transferred to Ward 5 on 29 July 2012 as is usual practice following initial assessment on the MAU. Staff noted that your mother remained drowsy. Intravenous antibiotics continued to be administered as prescribed.

Dr Jagus reviewed your mother on 31 July 2012 and noted the diagnosis of cholecystitis. Due to your mother's drowsiness, Dr Jagus discontinued the prescription of pregabalin and risperidone, and her diazepam was reduced from 5mgs to 2mgs three times a day. She was to continue to take Sodium Valproate 100mgs three times a day. Dr Jagus requested ward staff to liaise with Grianagh Court as to your mother's progress.

Your mother was reviewed by Dr Khuriajam on 02 August 2012. He requested a CT head scan due to your mother's continued drowsiness and her complaining of neck stiffness. A differential diagnosis of encephalitis or multiple strokes was made. If the scan was clear, the plan was to carry out a lumbar puncture to aid in diagnosis. Unfortunately, the CT scanner was out of action that day.

On 03 August your mother complained of leg pain. She was seen and examined by the on-call doctor, Dr Dale Saviour, F1 for Dr Balakrishnan. His examination found no swelling, all her pulses seemed normal and her legs were warm and well perfused. Dr Savoir prescribed paracetamol for the relief of this leg pain.

Your mother was reviewed by Dr Khuraijam, Locum Consultant Physician on 06 August 2012 and noted her observations, these being pulse, respirations and blood pressure were stable and that she did not have a temperature. There was concern over her poor oral intake and therefore the treatment plan was to insert a nasogastric tube to allow feeding to be administered over 16 hours a day, and to also give intravenous fluids. It is also documented that your mother was more awake, alert and consented to the nasogastric tube insertion. Dr Kharijam also requested that a date for the CT scan was obtained. Your mother was reviewed by the dietician and a feeding regime was drawn up.

On 07 August 2012, your mother was reviewed by Dr Majeed, Staff Grade Doctor, who noted that your mother was more alert, and that she denied any pain. The plan of nasogastric feeding, intravenous fluids and antibiotics was to continue.

On 08 August 2012, the CT scan was carried out and this showed cerebral atrophy, (but no change since the previous scan in 2010). Your mother remained drowsy and therefore the diazepam was reduced to 1mg twice a day.

On 11 August 2012, it was noted that your mother had removed her nasogastric tube. There was still concern that your mother was taking very little orally and therefore it was deemed necessary to insert a further nasogastric tube to continue with this method of feeding.

However, as the days progressed your mother became drowsy until on 13 August 2012 she would only open her eyes to painful stimuli. Dr Khuraijam discontinued the diazepam, mirtazapine and donepezil as he was aware that they could be a factor in her drowsiness. Further investigations including a repeat ultrasound scan of the abdomen, blood tests and MRI scan were also requested. Your mother removed her feeding tube once more and this was replaced by nursing staff as your mother was still not taking adequate food orally.

By the 14 August 2012, your mother was responding to vocal commands with spontaneous opening of her eyes.

On 15 August 2012, on his ward round. Dr Majeed reviewed

your mother's treatment and progress so far. The treatment plan was updated which was to include an MRI scan, surgical opinion, neurology opinion, continue with intravenous antibiotics and fluids, abdominal ultrasound scan and further urine samples to be obtained. A lumbar puncture was also carried out on 15 August 2012 which was unremarkable.

Your mother was reviewed by Dr. Khuriajam on 16 August 2012. He noted that your mother remained very drowsy but was more rousable. He noted that the Neurologist had not been able to examine your mother the previous day as she had been in the Radiology Department an undergoing MRI scan. The Neurologist had reviewed your mother's medical records and results from the lumbar puncture and had advised that staff continue to treat as an infection. Dr Khuriajam also noted the result of the MRI scan which were unremarkable.

On 20 August 2012 your mother was to be referred back to Grianagh Court for further care as she was much more alert, feeling better and responding to verbal commands, although she was still complaining of generalised tenderness in her abdomen. Your mother was reviewed by Dr Jagus on 21 August 2012. He noted that your mother was much more alert although she had become bed bound at that present time. He advised a gradual reduction of Sodium Valproate by 100mgs each dose time: medical staff agreed with this plan.

Over the next few days, your mother was reviewed by medical staff on a regular basis and they noted that she became more alert. Her nasogastric tube was removed, and nursing staff encouraged your mother to eat and drink. However, your mother became reluctant to take anything orally and therefore the possibility of inserting a Percutaneous Endoscopic Gastrostomy (PEG) feeding tube was discussed.

You, your husband and father met with Dr Kifayat Anwan, Staff Grade Doctor and Hannah Crawford, Dietician on 30 August 2012. This meeting was held to discuss the possibility of inserting the PEG feeding tube to ensure that your mother would receive the required fluid and nutrition support that she required. Dr Anwan advised that your mother, would need to be reviewed by the Psychiatrist before this procedure and that once this was done, a further meeting would be held with you all to discuss your mother's future care and treatment. Dr Anwan recalls that you enquired as to the possibility of your mother suffering from Neuroleptic Malignant Syndrome in the recent past. Dr Anwan explained that it was unlikely during this current admission and that the Psychiatrist would be the most appropriate person to speak to regarding this concern. Dr Anwan felt that he was unable to comment further as he had never met your mother prior to this admission.

Dr Anwan had documented that you understood your mother's condition very well, and that you requested a second opinion, asking that it would not be from Dr Jagus. You were reassured that staff would gladly meet anytime if concerns arose.

Your mother received ongoing monitoring for her health condition and the Dietician requested that the intravenous fluids were discontinued as your mother's nutritional requirements were to be met via her overnight feed. Her weight was monitored closely as staff identified that your mother was unable to receive sufficient intake, as she unfortunately persisted in pulling the nasogastric feeding tube out. It was believed that the best way forward would be to hold a multi-disciplinary meeting where it would be suggested that the PEG feeding tube was sited.

On 07 September 2012 Dr Majeed, Locum Staff Grade Doctor, Dr Jagus, Hannah Crawford, Dietician, Dr Seviar, Foundation Year 1 Doctor and a member of the nursing staff from Ward 5 met with you, your husband and your father. This meeting was recorded at your request and with the consent of the staff present. Dr Majeed explained about the infections that your mother had been treated for and about the various investigations that had been carried out. You raised the possibility of Neuroleptic Malignant Syndrome and Dr Jagus explained that it was unlikely. Dr Majeed explained that the issues of concern were your mother's drowsiness, her mobility and her nutritional intake. Dr Majeed advised that there did not appear to be a medical reason for her continued drowsiness and that the cause may never be identified. A discussion regarding a PEG tube being inserted took place and your family advised staff that you would consider this option. It was decided to continue with nasogastric feeding in the interim and a referral regarding the possibility of a PEG would be made to Dr Ashdown, Consultant Gastroenterologist.

Dr Jagus suggested an antidepressant (Mirtazapine) for your mother as this medication might improve your mother's appetite.

Over the next couple of weeks, the nasogastric tube was inserted on several occasions as your mother unfortunately continued to remove them. It was discussed and decided by Dr Majeed and Dr Seviar that the best option would be for the PEG to be inserted as soon as possible. A provisional date had originally been given for 21 September 2012. Dr Majeed contacted a doctor from the surgical team and requested earlier intervention.

Your mother was reviewed by Dr Mownah, Consultant Surgeon on the morning of 14 September 2012 who agreed that a PEG was a suitable option and arrangements were made to carry out the procedure under general anaesthetic. In the meantime, subcutaneous fluids were commenced to prevent dehydration and nursing staff encouraged your mother to take oral diet and fluids.

The procedure was due to be undertaken on 18 September 2012; however, this had to be postponed as blood tests revealed that your mother had a low potassium level. Replacement therapy was commenced, and the PEG was inserted on 20 September 2012.

Your mother was reviewed by the Dietician on 21 September 2012 and a feeding regime was commenced.

Unfortunately, on 23 September 2012, your mother began to suffer with vomiting and appeared to be in pain when fluid was flushed through the PEG. Your mother was seen and examined by Dr Muktadir, Surgical Senior House Officer on call. He discussed your mother with his senior, Mr Ratnavel, Associate Specialist, Surgery who advised that the PEG was not to be used overnight and to review again the following morning. Mr Mownah further reviewed your mother the following day and advised that fluids could be re-introduced via the PEG and increase as tolerated and advised by the Dietician. Mr Mownah also reviewed your mother the morning of 26 September 2012 where he noted cellulitis (inflammation of the skin) around the entry site of the PEG. He advised that the PEG site was to be covered to try and prevent your mother pulling at it and that the feed could be re-started.

The Nutritional Nurse Specialist and the Dietician also reviewed your mother later that day as she had begun to vomit again. Staff were advised that the PEG was not to be used and for your mother to be further reviewed by medical staff.

Mr Mownah was contacted and he arranged for a CT scan to be carried out to check the position of the PEG, as he suspected that your mother may have pulled at the tube and dislodged it. The CT scan showed that the tube was out of her stomach but reassuringly there were no signs of peritonitis. Intravenous fluids were to continue.

Dr Majeed met with you that evening and explained how poorly your mother was. Mr Mownah reviewed your mother the following morning and advised that the PEG was not to be used.

Dr Krishnan also met with you on 01 October 2012 to

explain that the surgeons were concerned about re-inserting a PEG, in that they believed that the risks to your mother outweighed the benefits. The advice was sought from the Dietician who documented that replacing the PEG would benefit your mother. The PEG tube was removed on 09 October 2012 and your mother was transferred to Ramsey and District Cottage Hospital on 15 October 2012, where she sadly passed away on 25 October 2012.

We hope now to be able to address your particular concerns.

Neuroleptic Malignant Syndrome

Neuroleptic Malignant Syndrome (NMS) is a condition that may occur as a serious complication of the use of anti-psychotic drugs. The exact incidence is difficult to calculate; however, it is very low. Whilst there are some clear risk factors, the low incidence and difficulties in studying the syndrome, the clinical features, predisposing conditions, treatment and prognosis are difficult to define.

The classic symptoms are that of severe muscular rigidity, significant hyperthermia (in particular malignant hyperthermia), autonomic instability and **changes in levels of consciousness**. Laboratory tests include raised **white cell count** and laboratory evidence of a muscle necrosis. Other clinical features which are present include **excessive sweating**, **difficulty swallowing**, **tremor**, **incontinence**, **delirium**, labile blood pressure, dyspnoea (shortness of breath), **psychomotor agitation**, severe muscle rigidity, **hyperthermia**, tachycardia, and a **shuffling gait**.

(Not in report, but*Bold* indicates symptoms that were reported in Judith's Mental Health records by a doctor or other staff members, on the first day of hospital admission, or the day prior to this).

In your mother's case it is not clear from your letter when you believe that the Neuroleptic Malignant Syndrome first began. Neuroleptic Malignant Syndrome is an acute complication, the severity of which peaks three days after onset, therefore Dr Jagus and

Dr Byrne, in the course of their investigation, presumed that you believe it occurred in the few days prior to your mother's admission to Noble's hospital on 20 July 2012.

Dr Jagus was on annual leave from 16 July 2012 to 20 July 2012 and was not present during this period of concern. His report and opinion are based only on reference to case records rather than personal contact with your mother at that time. As explained earlier, Dr Marie O'Sullivan was acting Locum during Dr Jagus' absence.

We feel that the best way forward therefore would be to structure the responses on Neuroleptic Malignant Syndrome by addressing specific points raised in your letter paragraph-by-paragraph.

In paragraph 2 of your letter you have written that you believe Dr Jagus failed in his duty to ensure that your mother was treated for Neuroleptic Malignant Syndrome alongside the infections that she was admitted to hospital for, and that urine infection and other infections can be a direct symptom of Neuroleptic Malignant Syndrome.

Dr Jagus was not on duty and was therefore unable to provide an opinion on whether your mother had Neuroleptic Malignant Syndrome or not. However, having reviewed the notes, symptoms and laboratory tests, these have shown no evidence that your mother was suffering from Neuroleptic Malignant Syndrome, although it would clearly always be in the differential diagnosis of somebody on antipsychotic drugs who became increasingly drowsy and developed pyrexia. At no point either, as far as Dr Jagus is aware, was it raised as a differential diagnosis by Noble's medical staff.

Severe muscle rigidity is one of the primary features of Neuroleptic Malignant Syndrome and on reviewing your mother's records; there is no documentation to suggest that she was demonstrating this. It is recorded that she was drowsy with poor mobility and certainly her physical examination by Dr Kjell-Arne Nordgard on the ward did not demonstrate any evidence of muscle rigidity.

Your mother was pyrexia, which is a feature of infection, but her temperature is not recorded as being higher than 38.5 degrees on 20 July 2012. Pyrexia in Neuroleptic Malignant Syndrome is often extremely high (up to 40 or 41 degrees) and is sometimes described itself as, "Malignant Hyperpyrexia" which needs specialist medical management in itself.

Regarding drowsiness and altered consciousness, we agree that this can be a feature of Neuroleptic Malignant Syndrome, but it is the opinion of the medical staff that it was more likely to be acute delirium caused by significant infection in a lady with pre-existing advanced dementia.

Your mother had a number of blood tests carried out on 20 July 2012 by Dr Kjell-Arne Nordgard. Her white blood cell count was raised which is an indicator of infection, although we agree that there can be leukocytosis (white blood cell count above normal range) present in Neuroleptic Malignant Syndrome, however it would be a rare differential diagnosis.

Her platelet count was normal at 274: however, thrombocytosis (high platelet count) is often present in Neuroleptic Malignant Syndrome. Her urea and electrolytes were entirely normal which would indicate no evidence of dehydration. Her bone profile including calcium was entirely normal. Hypocalcaemia (low calcium levels) is often a feature in Neuroleptic Malignant Syndrome and reassuringly, this was not present. Her liver function tests were very mildly deranged, however, based on the fact that she was known to have a very large gallstone, one would expect some disturbance of the liver function tests. On reviewing her case notes, it was noted that your mother had been known to have abnormal liver function tests since early 2011 and they had previously been more deranged than at this time.

As muscle necrosis is a classical feature of Neuroleptic Malignant Syndrome, certain blood tests including liver enzymes would be markedly raised as these are markers of muscle damage. We hope that we have been able to reassure you that the results of these investigations did not indicate the possibility of Neuroleptic Malignant Syndrome. There was no test for creatine kinase carried out at the time and this is characteristically very raised in Neuroleptic Malignant Syndrome, but this would probably only be tested had there been any suspicion at all that your mother was suffering from this condition. (Not in report. No urinalysis was undertaken to prove UTI or kidney infection).

In summary, as the timescale for Neuroleptic Malignant Syndrome is very acute, within one-to-three days, we have assumed during the course of this investigation that we are referring to the period prior to your mother's admission to Noble's Hospital, which is the period where it is alleged Neuroleptic Malignant Syndrome was missed. The absence of muscle rigidity, malignant hyperthermia and laboratory test profiles, which would indicate Neuroleptic Malignant Syndrome, demonstrates that as far as staff can ascertain from her records, there was no evidence of Neuroleptic Malignant Syndrome.

Neuroleptic Malignant Syndrome is a neurological condition which had a neurochemical basis and is not linked in any way to the likelihood of infection, which is clearly caused by infective organisms such as bacteria and viruses. Infection, however, was extremely likely to be the cause of the symptoms your mother presented with, particularly in view of the fact that she had dementia.

In paragraph 3 of your letter you advise that you noticed unusual muscle gain on your mother's legs on 30 May 2012 and that you believe this was a direct symptom of her developing Neuroleptic Malignant Syndrome

As mentioned above, the onset of Neuroleptic Malignant Syndrome is very acute over a short period, so this is not likely.

In paragraph four of your letter, you correctly indicate that your mother was being prescribed Diazepam, Risperidone and Mirtazapine together. Dr Jagus was asked to review your mother's medication history during this investigation. The mirtazapine had been a relatively longstanding medication which your mother had been taking for most of the period of her entire illness since 2008 because of the very high levels of depressive symptoms she presented with. Her risperidone was originally used, starting on 02 April 2012 by Dr Felix Nomuoja, Locum in Psychiatry, who admitted her to the ward on a section, as in her history noted above. Risperidone, in terms of evidence-base, has shown to be effective for aggressive behaviours in dementia, and ideally should be prescribed only for a period of six weeks for the behaviours in dementia. It has the best evidence-base of the atypical antipsychotic for this, however, it can be prescribed for longer periods of psychoses and mania. The clinical justification for this in your mother's case was that her aggression levels have been very high and whilst ward staff would endeavour to manage her in terms of her environment and their approach and their skills in de-escalating aggression, in some cases that are very high risk, it is necessary to continue the use of such medications. In addition, there are documented psychotic symptoms, so use of neuroleptic would be clinically appropriate. Dr Jagus reviewed all her psychotropic medications on 11 June 2012 and the risperidone was reduced along with some other psychotropic drugs being stopped and it was stopped altogether on 18 June 2012.

The risperidone was only re-started by Dr Marie O'Sullivan on 14 July 2012 and increased on 16 July 2012, again in response to aggressive and agitated behaviours; this demonstrated that your mother had only been on this medication for a maximum of six days prior to her admission and during the alleged period of Neuroleptic Malignant Syndrome. For some of this period it was withheld because she was so drowsy. The diazepam had been prescribed at 5mg three times a day by Dr Marie O'Sullivan on 30 June 2012, again because of significant problems with agitated and aggressive behaviours, including kicking and biting, and your mother had been on this since then and up to the point where she was admitted to Noble's Hospital. It is unlikely that diazepam could be implicated in Neuroleptic Malignant Syndrome as it is recognised as being amongst the many available treatments for Neuroleptic Malignant Syndrome itself. Although Dr Jagus was not present at the time, it is his opinion that it would appear that her drowsiness and change of mental state was due to an acute delirium due to her infection as mentioned above. Following review of your mother's healthcare records, Dr Byrne also agrees with this diagnosis.

In paragraph five of your letter, we note your concern regarding dehydration because of your mother's poor fluid intake. However, your mother's chemical pathology tests carried out on the ward, and also Noble's Hospital on her admission, were entirely normal with normal creatine and urea, which would not support a diagnosis of clinical dehydration.

We understand the concerns you raised in paragraph 6 in your letter with regard to the use of risperidone in dementia. We hope that we have been able to reassure you by the above that your mother was on this medication for a period of about two months because of her very high levels of aggression, but this was reviewed and it was only -re-started in the few days prior to her admission to Noble's Hospital. There were also psychotic symptoms present and therefore it is an appropriate treatment.

We do understand that it was distressing to see your mother develop a shuffling gait and becoming doubly incontinent. However, as we previously mentioned, there is a one-to-three day acute onset period of Neuroleptic Malignant Syndrome which, if it happened at all, could only have happened during the period prior to your mother's admission to Noble's Hospital rather than during her entire stay.

In paragraph 9 of your letter, you stated that Dr Jagus should have ensured that the neuroleptic drugs were withdrawn and treatment for Neuroleptic Malignant Syndrome started after its onset. As explained earlier, Dr Jagus was on annual leave at this point, and would not have been involved in this decision had Neuroleptic Malignant Syndrome been present in the first place. However, on reviewing your mother's records it is evident that staff believed that it was extremely likely that the symptoms your mother presented with were due to delirium secondary to infection and there would have been no particular reason to suspect Neuroleptic Malignant Syndrome, hence no clinical reason to stop the neuroleptic medications. The medication was reduced as your mother was drowsy.

In paragraph 10 of your letter, you have explained that you believe that the failure to treat the Neuroleptic Malignant Syndrome resulted in your mother becoming bedridden due to muscle necrosis, but please may we reassure you that there is no laboratory evidence on testing that muscle necrosis was present, and in particular, in view of her normal liver function test readings.

In paragraph 12 of your letter you state that two doctors on Ward 5 and Dr Jagus admitted that Neuroleptic Malignant Syndrome could have been a possibility "when pressed". In a meeting in Ward 5 on 07 September 2012, which Dr Jagus was involved in, he agreed that "could have been a possibility" but this is only based on the fact that it would always be amongst the differential diagnoses in the onset of a condition such as delirium, but in your mother's case the clinical features do not fit the diagnosis of Neuroleptic Malignant Syndrome.

Summary:-

In summary, although Dr Jagus was not present at work in the acute period leading up to your mother's admission to Noble's Hospital, from his perusal of her records, he believes there is no evidence that she was suffering for Neuroleptic Malignant Syndrome and was suffering from acute delirium caused by infection which was subsequently managed. Your mother's dementia has been a very unfortunate case with very distressing symptoms for both her and her family throughout the relatively short course of her illness, particularly in view of her relatively young age.

We do hope that this response helps to answer your concerns that you raised in your letter and at the meeting on 25 October 2012.

May we once again thank you for attending this meeting and for having the courage to speak so openly on what was a truly dreadful time for you.

Thank you for bringing these matters to our attention, we sincerely hope that we have fully addressed your concerns. We would like to assure you that it is our policy to do everything in our power to resolve complaints, although we also recognise that this is not always possible.

We aim to provide the best possible service to our patients and learning from these occasions when we fall short helps us to do better in the future. If, having read our response, you feel a meeting would be beneficial to clarify any residual issues arising out of your complaint, please do not hesitate to contact Tony Warham, Patient Safety and Governance Manager on 650793, who would be pleased to make the necessary arrangements. If you do not wish for such a meeting to take place, or we have not heard from you by 21 January 2013, we will assume that Local Resolution has concluded and we will close your file.

If you are dissatisfied with our response to your complaint you have the right to request, within twenty-eight days, consideration of your complaint by the Independent Review Body. Should you wish to exercise this right, you should write to them on or before 18 January 2013. Their address is-

Independent Review Body
PO Box 281
Douglas
Isle of Man
IM99 2SH

Please provide them with the following information-

Patient's name
Patient's address
Patient's date of birth
The date of receipt of this letter
A full account of your complaint and why you remain dissatisfied with the outcome of Local Resolution.
Yours sincerely

Barbara Scott
Hospital Manager

Steve Chell
Head of Mental Health Services

24
True Colours

I had now received some of Judith's medical notes from the Mental Health Unit. They insisted that my father sign the request and we had to go in person to collect them, with my father present. Could they be any more awkward if they tried? I had to physically help my father into my car and drive him all the way to their unit in Douglas. Meet with some random woman and collect the records – many of which were unsurprisingly missing.

I flicked through the records and realised that in order to process the information, I was going to need a full day to re-organise the material into some kind of order. (I noted that a copy of Dr. Jagus' holiday roster was included).

Before that though, I wished to address the report letter, that I had just received from the hospital. I rang Amanda Mills, Case Manager and explained that I had further issues with the letter. She asked me to forward the concerns my e-mail, which I proceeded to do:-

"14 December 2012

Dear Amanda
Further to our telephone conversation and the report that I received, I have made the following observations and have the following concerns:-

My first instance of raising my concerns over my mother's

swelling in her face and arms was made to Margaret Quayle (should have been Halsall), at Grianagh Court. I pressed around my mother's face and neck, in front of her and said that this was what I was really worried about. It looked like an adverse drug reaction to her medication.

The second incident of raising the swelling issue that I recall, was upon my mother being discharged back to Grianagh Court when the doctor clad in motorcycle gear, bar his helmet, visited my mother in her room. Delia, my mother's named assigned nurse present too.

The third incident was at her admission to the Medical Assessment Unit, when I spoke to the doctor wearing the hijab, who I now believe to be Dr. Ibrahim. I specifically explained that I was concerned about the swelling and stiffness around her face and neck. The doctor felt around my mother's neck and face while I was there. Dr Ibrahim then asked me how they were to get a urine sample from my mother.

Surely, raising these issues must be documented?

At no point during these three incidents of explaining my concerns over the swelling/solidness was I aware of Neuroleptic Malignant Syndrome, or of the drugs that my mother was being prescribed.

In Ward 5, as previously explained (some weeks after her first admission to Noble's), I was made aware of the drug, Risperidone, that my mother was taking. At this point I looked up the side-effects of this medication and was astonished by the swelling and mental-alertness issues associated with the side-effect known as Neuroleptic Malignant Syndrome, linked to the taking of risperidone.

At this point and further reading, I knew that my mother was likely to die, as a result of it remaining undetected for so long. I detailed this in my first letter to Grianagh Court.

Dr Jagus, in his first meeting, that I have recorded, and Dr Byrne, in the second meeting attended by yourself, assured me that my mother had not taken Risperidone since being admitted to Noble's. Dr Jagus said this was due to drowsiness and Dr Byrne said it had completely been withdrawn on 20 July. Both statements are incorrect as detailed in my mother's records, and a blatant untruth.

I believe that Dr Jagus was my mother's Consultant Psychiatrist, despite Dr. O'Sullivan being Locum while he was on annual leave, therefore I still consider it Dr Jagus' responsibility to oversee my mother's condition, after being admitted to Noble's, and being overly sedated by drugs prescribed under his medical supervision.

I understand that the use of risperidone in elderly dementia patients is highly monitored for side-effects and that risperidone is classed as a "black triangle" drug by the MHRA, due to its life-threatening side-effects, when used in these circumstances.

I noted your comments on the delirium. When my mother was admitted to Noble's she was well beyond a state of severe delirium, but I expect part of the treatment for that would be to withdraw any delirium-inducing medication too, alongside any infection. As mentioned previously, nobody was aware of the issues surrounding my mother's altered, incapacitated state, at Ward 1 and 2. They were only aware of the issue of the infection, when I brought the issue of incapacitation up. Presumably, nobody from Grianagh Court informed them on hand-over, of the serious altered state of consciousness. Delirium superimposed on dementia can be brought on by antipsychotic, sedatives, benzodiazepines and hypnotic-sedatives, I believe and by urinary tract infections too – always a possible issue surely, when doubly incontinent. Delirium prevention must be called for in these circumstances or at the very least, early recognition of the signs. Again, I must re-iterate that she was in an assessment unit for older mentally ill patients.

There are competency issues, both medically and in this

whole process, along with Mental Health Act 1998 issues and basic Human Rights issues.

My mother's death was a torturous affair for her, and her family witnessing it. From a hospital aspect it was incredibly expensive – over twelve weeks long. Mistakes have been made and attitudes are complacent. She was then put on the Liverpool Care Pathway, after all this.

Her Death Certificate reads as, "Dementia and Essential Hypertension".

In conclusion, I personally think that my mother's body was struggling with an infection and struggling to process all the medication that she was on because of it, but just for good measure, she was inappropriately given Risperidone to totally incapacitate her. Then just to double check that there was no possibility of recovering, the specialist psychiatric drugs were not removed when they critically need to be.

Yours sincerely
Victoria Quine"

I perused the report numerous times and re-read literature on Neuroleptic Malignant Syndrome. Other issues were immensely profound that I needed to raise further. Therefore, a second e-mail was sent to Amanda:-

"16 December 2012
Supplemental to the previous document attachment of 14 December and sent to Amanda Mill's e-mail address.

After having more time to read through the case report, I now have some further questions and point to raise.

Firstly, I believe that Risperidone causes extra-pyramidal signs, one of which I believe can be a feeding disorder, which clearly my mother was suffering from since her over-sedation in Grianagh Court.

Her urinary tract infections were addressed pretty quickly, so I believe that she was highly unlikely to die from these.

Apart from dementia which I'm led to believe was in the early stages, (although accompanied by the aggression and severe behavioural problem), the dementia was nowhere near the life-threatening stages likely to kill her. In the meeting recorded on 07 September, Dr Jagus described my mother as having "the early onset of dementia".

I knew that something about my mother's case was not right. Straight from seeing her overly sedated, followed by the blown-up, solid swelling around her face and neck, along with the noticeable pallor. Nothing is adding up in my opinion.

I would like to know when her temperatures were high, especially during her first admission to Ward 1 and 2.

I note from the Nitrofurantoin dosage, 250mg four times daily. Is this not a very unusually high dosage, especially knowing that she had abnormal liver function test since 2011, as detailed in the case report?

Could somebody please explain why my mother was on Pregablin, which I note was withdrawn on 31 July by Dr Jagus, along with risperidone and diazepam. Again, I note that Pregablin should be used with caution when used with other sedative drugs. Was any caution used at all – my mother was taking Risperidone, Mirtazapine, Diazepam and pregabalin together? Were these being used to treat her or kill her?

I note that side-effects of Nitrofurantoin are dizziness; drowsiness; dry mouth; increased creatine kinase levels which can cause muscle injury – coincidentally another side-effect of Neuroleptic Malignant Syndrome. Why was my mother given this medication when she had a history of B12 deficiency? I believe that side-effects of this can lead to symptoms of anorexia or feeding problems too?

Could liver function abnormality actually impair the hepatic metabolism of Risperidone as well as Nitrofurantoin?

I am totally amazed that Dr Jagus did not visit my mother in hospital until 31 July 2012. The drug combinations astound me as a lay-person. He knows the possible consequences of his prescribing them to her.

I also wish to know what happened after Delia, my mother's named nurse at Grianagh Court rang me at home, on my landline and asked me if I still wanted a meeting with Dr Jagus, after my mother had been admitted to Noble's hospital. I specifically said that I did, but no further contact with me was made. Determining what happened to this is really important to me, as this meeting could have resolved certain concerns about my mother's condition. A bin bag of clothes was dropped into the ward by Delia, but no further communication about this meeting. Dr Jagus would have returned from annual leave at this point.

I think it needs to be highlighted that my mother was in the Assessment Unit when she became incapacitated, firstly through over-sedation and then I suspect through an adverse reaction to medication that she was being prescribed whilst there, which I strongly believe led to the ultimate cause of her death.

All the drugs prescribed to her at the time explicitly detail that caution is required when being prescribed with other sedative drugs. There doesn't appear to have been any caution, whatsoever, demonstrated in my mother's case. Something has desperately gone wrong I believe.

Please rest assured that I am not pursuing this case for any financial gain or claim. I am extremely concerned that other vulnerable dementia patients are in danger.

I hope that these concerns can be addressed either during a meeting or by written correspondence".

25
The Grieving

Just before Christmas my father decided to book himself onto a coach trip in Scotland for Christmas. He explained that he couldn't bear to stay on the island for Christmas without Judy. And in his words, "all that happiness and hugging and kissing". He was so sad and miserable. He did nothing to try and hide the fact. Without trying to sound harsh, ten minutes in his company was enough to drag anybody to the depths of despair too. There was no other way to feel about it. If you care for somebody who is having a seriously depressing time, it is almost impossible not to feel their pain too. I knew how desperately sad and lonely he was since Judith's death, but the, "I am going to kill myself", over the telephone at night-time was wearing me down too. I was trying to stay positive, but it was a constant battle. I dreaded how people in his company on a coach trip, for Christmas especially, would deal with him.

We all told him that it was a very bad idea. He had already suffered a stroke and if something happened to him up in the highlands, he might be completely alone and stranded. Actually, he said that he didn't care if he died there. Jesus!! I reluctantly offered to go with him, but he insisted that he wanted to go alone, and might even pick up a lady friend. His previous stroke had left him with a profound lack of sensitivity and devoid of empathy. I had never seen him like this before.

He was going for just five days and returning on Boxing day. I had hoped that he would come to his senses before Christmas arrived, but he did not. He had booked and paid for his seat at the front of the coach. He had arranged a door to door taxi over to Liverpool to catch the coach, and back. Jim's sister, Muriel, rang me with her concerns about him travelling to Scotland for Christmas, but she had attempted to persuade him not to go, and had failed miserably too. We all tried our utmost to persuade Jim that he was making a bad decision, but he was not having any of it. We had told him that, not only was he vulnerable with his mobility, but that he would be desperately lonely too.

Not to be swayed, he departed for his trip. His mobility was really not good, and he would be unable to climb on and off the coach by himself. I was assured by the coach trip organisers that he would be assisted. My father rang me, or I rang him, every day. Sadly, he didn't seem to be enjoying his trip at all. He really disliked some of the people, and a couple of times when he had told people that he had recently lost his wife; they had told him that he should be back in the Isle of Man with his family.

On Christmas Day, my father rang in tears. Sophie, Chris and Roly, along with his girlfriend were all at our house. My poor father was desperately lonely and missing Judy. He had fallen out with one gentleman, who had asked my father why he had even bothered to come on the coach trip, as he told Jim that he was trying to make everybody as miserable as he was feeling. This gentleman refused to sit next to Jim for Christmas lunch and therefore my father had sat by himself. I wanted to cry for him too. My heart was breaking for him. He was in such a black hole and appeared to be digging himself even deeper. Sometime after Judy had died, Jim had gone to his G.P. for some antidepressants, but they clearly had no beneficial effect on Jim. Thankfully he was due back the next day, later in the evening. I had asked him to ring me when he returned home.

On Boxing Day, he rang me to say that he had arrived back at his house. I was so relieved. Nigel and I drove over to see him, bringing a food parcel too. We arrived outside his bungalow and rang the doorbell, before walking straight in, as my father's walking was too bad for him to get up in any haste. When I saw him, I must have looked shocked. He appeared so, so frail and ill. His eyes looked glassy and he looked exhausted too. I put some lights on as he was in the near dark. I lit the gas fire for him, then made us all a drink. Nigel started chatting with Jim while I made the tea.

It transpired that my father had hated almost everything about the trip – the long journey; the coach driver; the woman who was sitting next to him; all of the hotels and most of the food. He really was at the lowest ebb I had ever seen him. His suitcase was on the floor of the lounge, probably where the taxi driver had left it. After our tea, I said that I would unpack it for him. He told me to leave it, but I explained that it was no trouble for me. Then he shouted, "I told you to leave it, now bloody leave it". I backed off and asked if he wanted me to heat his dinner, but he informed me that he was so tired and just wanted to go to bed. I let him know that his meal was in the fridge, if he did want it later. I hugged my father and asked if there was anything I could do for him. "Give me a shotgun", was his reply. I was desperately sorry for my father; I had no answers to relieve his mental anguish and torment.

I visited my father every other day, and Sophie visited in the evenings after work. He really was just existing, and in a really unpleasant place in his head: he was deeply depressed. I was therefore very surprised when he insisted on driving to our house on New Year's Day, and actually seemed enthusiastic about doing so too. We would go to our usual place for New Year's Day, the Creg-ny-Baa. Nigel had offered to go and get Jim from Ramsey, but my father insisted he could drive over. Sophie and Chris were coming over too, but still he wanted to drive himself. So, on New Year's Day, as normal, Kana the dog jumped up, as she heard Jim's car coming down the country lane. Sophie and Chris were already at our house by this point.

My father reversed into the driveway, as he usually did, only this time he kept reversing until he hit my 2CV car. We were all a little shocked but didn't make a big deal about it; almost as if it never happened, although Nigel intervened and shouted for him to stop reversing.

I walked over to help him get out of the car. His face was greyer than I had ever seen it, and his eyes were so glassy-looking again. We all went into the lounge and I couldn't help but show my concern. I had asked him if he felt fine in himself and then told him that I was seriously concerned about him, as he looked most unwell. He was a little irritated by this, so I apologised, hugged him and we all took turns in wishing him a Happy New Year. I asked him if he still wanted to go out for a meal at the Creg, but he explained that he was in fact not hungry now. I informed him that he didn't need to go there, and that I could cancel or postpone the meal. It wasn't an issue. Yet my father decided that he would still attend and have perhaps a smaller meal.

We drove the ten minutes up there, in Nigel's and Chris' car, with my father in with us. We sat in our normal window seat in the restaurant looking out to Douglas Bay. We ordered our drinks and Jim decided that he would have a brandy and coke, explaining that he had not taken a drink for a year. It was only a single measure, so it wouldn't affect his driving. Although I was already considering asking him to travel back with Chris and Sophie in their car. He did seem perkier in himself, but seriously looked like death warmed up.

After the meal and returning to our house, my father wished to drive back to Ramsey immediately. I suggested that he go with Sophie and Chris, but he rejected the idea.

After he had left, we all agreed that he looked absolutely terrible. Sophie and Chris would go back soon after and visit him at his bungalow, to ensure that he got back safely. Sophie rang me later to confirm that he was back at home, but she said that he looked even worse than he had earlier. I was just thankful that he was home.

The following morning, I received a telephone call at around 10 a.m. At first, I thought it was a prank caller, as I could not hear anybody at the other end of the line, but then my heart sank, as I heard my father's slow drawl. It seemed, from what I could understand, that he had fallen in the bathroom during the night and had lain there for some hours before he had managed to crawl to the bedroom. All I think that I said was, "I am coming now", then threw down the phone and shouted to Nigel that I was going to Ramsey. As I explained the circumstance to him, Nigel got his coat and drove us over to Ramsey. He was a much quicker driver than me. It perhaps took us only twenty minutes to get there. The mountain road has no mandatory speed limit, so a clear road was an open road. Luckily Nigel had remembered the spare keys to my father's house, so we were able to let ourselves in. I rushed into my father's bedroom and saw him lying there helplessly. My immediate reaction was to hug and kiss him. His speech was slurred and his pupil in one eye looked dilated. I immediately rang for an ambulance.

My father tried to explain, as best he could, that he had fallen when he went to the bathroom during the night. He had felt dizzy and lost consciousness he thought. He had not managed to get up when he had come around, and he felt like he had stayed there for hours and had become very cold. Eventually he had managed to crawl to the bedroom and somehow into bed. He had clearly pulled his bedside locker over in attempting this, as the contents were scattered around the bedroom floor.

When the ambulance arrived with the paramedic and the technician, they asked me to explain what had happened. They then went into my father's bedroom and asked him various questions, like his name, his date of birth, how many fingers were they holding up. They then came out and explained that it was probably a urine infection, as quite often elderly people would fall over going to the bathroom when they had such an infection. I disagreed and explained that I thought it was a stroke, or a seizure as he had suffered with them before.

They decided that the best plan of action would be to take Jim to Ramsey and District Cottage Hospital for a check-up. I informed them that I would follow in the car.

When we arrived at the hospital, the crew put my father in a wheelchair and sat him in the reception area with me. We were called into a doctor's room by a lady, who explained that we would be seeing, "the baby doctor". I was a little confused. Seeing that, she explained that the new doctor they had looked so young that she was fondly called, "baby doctor".

The doctor arrived sometime after. She was quite young, immediately looked like a hockey player to me – a little bit boyish with short hair and a tomboy air about her. She seemed polite and was friendly with me. She was asking my father questions, and when he answered them as best he could, she was almost shouting at him, making him most flustered. Maybe this was a good approach she thought, but either way, she just came across as impolite and intimidating to me. After a serious amount of questions, pulling arms, and counting fingers, it was decided to place my father in a ward for the night, for observation.

Afterwards he was taken on to the ward and I returned to his house to collect some pyjamas and toiletries for him. I explained that I would return as soon as I had collected them. Nigel was waiting at my father's house. There had seemed little point in both of us going with Jim. Nigel had kindly sorted the house and washed the bedding and cleaned the bathroom up too.

We both drove out to buy some lunch, which we ate back at my father's house. After lunch and a coffee, I returned to the ward to see my father and deliver his belongings. He had in the meantime recognised some of the staff from when Judith was in there. Everybody was sympathetic with him and he seemed to be enjoying the attention.

Later on, I kissed him goodbye and explained that I would return the next day. I felt relieved to know that my father was being looked after and that he would be warm and comfortable.

The next morning, I rang the ward to see how my father was overnight. I spoke with a nurse, who explained that Jim was sitting up in bed and seemed very bright. I asked her to please let him know that I would visit in a few hours. After putting the phone down, I felt a little happier, knowing he looked perkier.

Only moments later the phone rang, which I answered. It was

the nurse who I had just spoken with. Her first words were, "I am so sorry". My heart hit the floor.

She continued to explain that after she had spoken with me, she went to speak with Jim. He wasn't in his bed, so she went in search of him. She found him lying on the floor in the bathroom, collapsed. They had called an ambulance and they were taking him straight to Noble's hospital.

I asked her how he had ended up in the bathroom. She replied that he had gotten there himself. But wasn't he under observation, and were the bed sides not up, I asked? She said that she was so sorry, but they were not.

Ok, what had happened had happened, I told myself. We couldn't change that. I tried to remain calm. I asked her to please ring me when he had left in the ambulance for Noble's. She did just that when the ambulance departed with Jim.

I waited for half an hour and then drove with Nigel to Noble's Hospital. After reaching the hospital and asking for directions at reception, we got to Jim's Ward. He was lying in bed, very confused when we arrived, and unable to string a sentence together. He had a cardboard-type bowl by him and was feeling sick. Evidence on the bed sheets told us he had been sick. The nurse came over and explained that they were doing various tests on him including CT and MRI scans. While we were there, the porters came to collect Jim for tests. My father had to be physically lifted from the bed to the wheelchair, and they then strapped him in. My father was attempting to ask questions but could not manage more than one drawn-out word. The nurse asked us to come back later, after all the tests had been done. They would update us then.

I could barely comprehend the series of events, but firstly, I needed to return to Ramsey and collect my father's belongings again, to take when I visited him later that evening.

I collected my father's things later from his house and the previous hospital ward, then dropped by to my father's next door neighbour's, to let them know what was going on. They kept an eye on Jim and might have been concerned to see no lights on in his house.

Later that evening, myself and Nigel returned to the Ward to check on my father and his results. Before we got to my father, the Sister of the Ward asked to have a word with us. She went on to explain that Jim had suffered a subarachnoid haemorrhage in the brain. He was critically ill and under normal circumstances, they would fly him across to Liverpool for surgery, but his condition was too serious for the flight over, and he probably would not even survive the flight. She then went on to explain that the last fall was the most likely cause for the haemorrhage. The next forty eight hours were critical. If the bleeding continued, then he would probably die as a result. The nurse looked panic stricken and I felt that she was searching my face for some reaction to this information. She clearly had no idea of what I had recently experienced with my mother. Nothing shocked me now. My expectations were very low. She must have thought that I was very nonchalant and calm even. In my head I was cursing a thousand times over. I understood his condition, I said and the severity of it. I went to see my father on the ward. He was immensely confused and tired. He had an, "assisted feeding" notice above his bed.

We sat with him talking in general and assisted him with taking a drink. He could not raise his hands to his mouth at this point.

Thankfully, the bleed appeared to have stopped by the third day. We didn't really know how much brain damage he may have suffered, but they would probably move my father to the Rehabilitation Ward, in perhaps one weeks' time. From the condition of my father, this was going to be a very long recovery, if indeed he would make it at all.

Sophie and I were still desperately affected by Judith's death. Travelling to the hospital everyday again, was like reliving the events once more. Just setting foot back into the hospital was difficult.

26
The Unearthing

My next correspondence from the hospital with regards to Judith, was dated 29 January 2013. The letter was extensive:-

> "Dear Mrs Quine
> Thank you for your e-mails dated 14 and 16 December 2012. This was following our response letter dated 11 December 2012. We are sorry that after receiving this response you have been left with unresolved issues. We forwarded your residual concerns to the Mental Health Service and also the Managers of the Medical and Surgical Divisions at Noble's Hospital and we are now able to offer the following information:-

Paragraphs 1 – 4

Doreen Fell, Senior Practitioner at Grianagh Court has reviewed your mother's records and has noted on 20 July 2012 your mother had become extremely drowsy. She was on duty at that time with Registered Nurse (RN) Halsall (not Quayle). Dr Nordgard was requested to review your mother. Dr Nordgard has recorded at 15:16 hours that he was asked to review your mother as she was drowsy ad had developed a rash on her legs. He noted your mother's temperature as 37.4 degrees Celsius and that she was drowsy. On examining your mother, he noted that your mother had a dry tongue and mucous membranes. There was no leg swelling, but a rash on both shins was noted. Her heart sounds were regular and her lungs seemed clear on auscultation. Her abdomen was soft, but she appeared to be tender in her left flank.

Dr Nordgard's clinical differential diagnosis was a fever of unknown origin, and dehydration. The possible diagnosis of pyelonephritis was given as your mother was currently on Nitrofurantoin for a urinary tract infection. No neck or facial swelling was noted at the time. Your father was present at this time. RN Halsall attempted to assist your mother in taking fluids, but she was **unable to swallow**. Mrs Fell has confirmed that your mother's neck was not swollen at the time.

Later that afternoon, R.N. Halsall noticed your mother's **neck was swollen**. You were also present and your mother was waiting to be transferred to Noble's hospital. In reviewing your mother's records, we are able to confirm that no medication had been administered to your mother for twenty four hours.

On 28 July 2012 at 1617 hours R.N. Dela Rosa asked the duty doctor to review your mother. R.N. Dela Rosa was concerned about your mother's overall condition. Dr Ziajka attended the ward and examined your mother. Your mother was transferred to the Medical Assessment Unit (MAU) at Noble's Hospital. It was at this point that HCA Moore noticed your mother's **neck was swollen**.

Your mother was admitted to the MAU at Noble's Hospital and was seen and examined by Dr Ibrahim at 1600 hours. Your mother's temperature was recorded as 37.00 degrees Celsius. The rash on her shins was noted and it was noted that there was no oedema (swelling). There is no documentation specifically mentioning swelling at this point. Neck stiffness is first recorded on 02 August 2012, during Dr Khurijam's (Locum Consultant Physician) Ward round. A CT scan was arranged.

Paragraph 5
With regards to Neuroleptic Malignant Syndrome again, as covered in the extensive first report we provided, there was no clinical evidence that your mother ever had Neuroleptic Malignant Syndrome.

Paragraph 6
This mentions Neuroleptic Malignant Syndrome but again, there is no evidence that this was the case.

Paragraph 7

This paragraph suggests that Neuroleptic Malignant Syndrome had remained undetected for a significant period of time, but as we covered in our previous response, the condition is an acute clinical state which peeks after 3 days, so this could not have been present for weeks or months.

Paragraph 8

Further to you raising this concern, Dr Jagus re-examined the medications chart from your mother's healthcare records at the time of her first admission to Noble's Hospital on 20 July 2012. It would appear that you are correct and the Risperidone was not stopped on admission to Noble's Hospital. On a Medical Ward, medications regime would normally be reviewed by the admitting medical team and medications continued or stopped as felt appropriate. Dr Jagus has reviewed the medical card which was in place during your mother's admission in Grianagh Court, which was transferred over to Noble's Hospital with her and runs until 26 July 2012. He is able to confirm that your mother did actually have a number of doses of Risperidone 0.5mgs during these first few days, but also notes that there were a majority of occasions where it was prescribed where it was not administered to her because the chart indicates it was either not available or your mother was asleep or drowsy. There is a subsequent drug chart which dates from 27 July 2012 which was written by one of the doctors at Noble's Hospital and they have continued all of the medication as prescribed.

However, the risperidone was not administered at all according to this drug chart, as were a majority of all other medications. Dr Jagus then stopped the medication on 31 July 2012 when he reviewed your mother at Noble's Hospital. Having re-examined the drugs charts, Dr Jagus has realised that his suggestion that the medication was completely stopped on admission was an error on his part and he would seek to assure you that this was not a blatant untruth. He truly did not set out to deceive you. (Not in report, but, is it really acceptable for a Consultant Psychiatrist to "not know", that his patient, had a review by another Psychiatrist from the same unit, after the patient had been transferred from the Mental Health Unit, and to "not know", that all medication had been continued, in spite of a "danger of polypharmacy", being written in Judith's notes, by another Psychiatrist's input).

Paragraph 9

We note that you believe that Dr Jagus should have retained clinical responsibility over your mother once she was transferred to Noble's Hospital. We would like to explain that whilst your mother remained under Dr Jagus, once transferred to a Ward at Noble's Hospital, clinical responsibility and decisions over investigations, medication and treatment rest with the Consultant managing her at that stage and it is not routine practice for a patient to be automatically reviewed by whichever clinician she had been transferred from. Your mother was under the care of Mr Mownah, Locum Consultant Surgeon, from 20-27 July 2012 and then from 28 July 2012 onwards, having been transferred back to Grianagh Court for one day over the intervening weekend.

Paragraph 10 and 11

You are correct regarding the general concerns there have been in medical practice recently, over the use of Risperidone and other antipsychotic medication in Dementia. These concerns are well justified by evidence, but concern only the treatment of agitation rather than the behavioural and psychiatric symptoms in dementia (BPSD), such as depression, aggression and psychotic symptoms such as hallucinations and delusions, which can be highly distressing.

There is evidence that risperidone can be beneficial for aggression (rather than agitation), but it is also an antipsychotic and in the presence of psychotic symptoms such as hallucinations, it would still be considered an appropriate treatment, even in patients with dementia. Indeed, in documents such as the Royal College of Psychiatrists (e.g. Atypical Antipsychotics and Behavioural and Psychiatric Symptoms in Dementia), with regard to this. It clearly states that antipsychotic drugs should still be used where there is a specific indication such as psychosis, "Drugs may be an appropriate first response to BPSD symptoms in the following situations: where drugs have a specific indication, (e.g. depression or psychosis), whatever the severity and frequency of the symptom".

We know from your mother's presentation that as well as a high level of aggressive symptoms, she did have psychotic symptoms such as hallucinations and delusional ideas, accompanied by very high levels of distress to herself and it would therefore be deemed appropriate to treat her with medication such as Risperidone at the small doses which she was taking, but keep this under review. The Risperidone was initially stopped approximately 8 weeks after it was started by Dr Nomuoja in April 2012.

Paragraph 12

This paragraph refers again to Neuroleptic Malignant Syndrome, but I reiterate that there is no evidence clinically that it was present. The Risperidone was recommended just prior to the episode in question by Dr O'Sullivan due to a resurgence in symptoms of agitation and aggression.

Paragraph 13

This paragraph refers to your mother being bedridden just prior to her admission to Noble's hospital and following this. Again, from experience, this would fit with severe delirium superimposed on dementia as this often causes alterations in consciousness and changes in mobility.

Paragraph 14

On reviewing your mother's healthcare records on RiO, the Mental Health Service electronic records, it is noted that your mother first refused a meal on the evening 18 July 2012, although she accepted lunch on 19 July 2012. Previous to this, your mother had taken what staff assessed to be good amounts of diet and fluids.

Paragraph 15

Further to paragraph 9 above, we acknowledge your comments which suggest that Dr Jagus should have visited your mother immediately on the medical ward following his return from leave. On returning Dr Jagus was informed that she had been admitted to Noble's with pyelonephritis and was physically unwell and being treated with intravenous antibiotics. At this stage, Dr Jagus did not feel it appropriate to visit her as her clinical care at that point was resting with the Consultant in charge of her medical care at Noble's Hospital. Staff at Noble's Hospital are aware that they can contact the Mental Health Service at any time for advice and support.

During the weekend, your mother was transferred back to Grianagh Court and then back to Noble's again; this time to be treated for cholecystitis. Dr Jagus chose then to visit her on 31 July 2012 to review medication and his contact with her at this stage is recorded in Noble's notes. Dr Jagus had not been requested to visit her but felt it would be appropriate just to maintain contact from our service with the medical team. (Not in report, but, this is untrue. Medics requested a Psychiatric review on 30 July).

Paragraph 16

A urine sample was taken on 12 July 2012, whilst your mother was still under the care of Grianagh Court. This confirmed the presence of an infection and Nitrofurantoin was prescribed. On your mother's admission to Ward 1 no further urine sample was taken as an infection had been identified 8 days earlier. Medical staff discussed your mother's blood results, urine tests and clinical findings with Dr Anson, Consultant Microbiologist, Royal Liverpool University Hospital who advised that Gentamycin was commenced and Nitrofurantoin should be discontinued. There were two further urine samples taken during your mother's time in Noble's Hospital. The first was 16 August 2012, as a routine due to the fact that your mother by this stage had a catheter in situ. No infection was present at that time. The second was on 14 September 2012 where an infection was identified. (Not in report, but, seeing as no urinalysis was performed on her admission to the medical ward on 20 July, the UTI or kidney infection was a clinical diagnosis only).

Paragraph 17 and 18

In these paragraphs we note your concern that we are suggesting that you mother was very frail and that this was the possible reason why infection may have resulted in her death. We would like to reassure you that this was not the case, Dr Jagus was not of the opinion that she was physically frail overall. Dr Jagus recalls that your mother had always been a relatively young and generally physically fit lady whose primary problems were the cognitive and mental effects of her dementia. Both Dr Jagus and the rest of the team involved in your mother's care believe that it was her frail physical state which resulted in her demise. (Conflicting statements here).

Dr Jagus is of the opinion that she developed severe and acute delirium superimposed on her dementia as a result of infection. Epidemiological studies show mortality rates in dementia in hospitalised patients to be very high and up to 76% in some studies. Even following treatment of the delirium, the one-year mortality rate is 35-40%. Delirium can also be prolonged even after the treatment of the underlying causes such as infection and the hypoactive form of delirium can result in continued impairment of conscious levels and continued symptoms of delirium. He is of the opinion that this was the case in Mrs Allen's situation following the treatment of the cholecystitis, where she remained drowsy and poorly responsive for some time. We are aware that your mother was investigated for conditions such as encephalitis, but it is likely that her presentation was due to prolonged hypoactive delirium.

Paragraph 19

We note that you believe that risperidone had caused her incontinence. However, incontinence is a recognised and very frequent symptom of advancing dementia. When your mother was admitted to Grianagh Court in 2011, staff noted that she was incontinent at times. Staff were able to direct her and assist her to manage. They also noted that she was prone to urinary infections.

Staff recall that as your mother's dementia progressed and worsened, she unfortunately became doubly incontinent and she needed to wear incontinence pants. Your mother would at times shred these pants and staff sometimes found it challenging to help her as she became agitated and aggressive at times on occasions, biting and kicking staff. Mrs Fell would like to offer her apologies if you believe that the pants were too tight. It was never their intention to cause any more distress or anxiety to your mother and her family.

Dr Jagus, as your mother's Consultant believes that her dementia was advanced as she had had it for a number of years and believes it is very likely that the increase in symptoms such as incontinence of urine and faeces were due to her advancing dementia rather than specifically due to Risperidone. (Not in report, but, the incontinence issues only started in the period between April 2012 to July 2012, whilst she was in Grianagh Court).

Paragraph 20

It would not be appropriate to automatically inform relatives of medical details or medication because as we are sure you will appreciate, confidentiality issues may prevent this. However, Dr Jagus had been managing your mother's dementia since 2008 and would always see and discuss things with her relatives if they requested this. He undertakes a weekly ward round on the ward and is always amenable to speaking to relatives if they request this, so there would have been ample opportunity for you to meet with him if they wished to discuss which medication she was taking and the reasons for this. We understand that your father came into the ward almost every day and it is reported that he had numerous discussions with staff regarding her care. (Not in report, but, Dr Jagus had the responsibility to inform us, as relatives, about the medication, especially risperidone, with its risks and benefits, especially when prescribed with furosemide and the "danger of polypharmacy", noted in Judith's Mental Health records. He chose not to do this).

Paragraph 21

We totally understand your concerns about the use of antipsychotic in dementia because this is a practice which has been controversial and prominent in the press in recent years, However, we believe that we acted appropriately in the treatments that we gave and as outlined below, staff were doing their best to manage a very difficult case of Alzheimer's Disease, particularly characterised by very high levels of distress and psychotic symptoms and agitation and aggression which, for your mother, must have been extremely unpleasant and distressing. One term used to describe her mental state by staff on occasions was "tortured" and obviously in this type of condition, we need to do our best to alleviate this and give patients some peace of mind and quality of life if possible.

We will now address your concerns raised in your e-mail dated 16 December 2012 and as before, address each paragraph in turn.

Paragraph 1

Extra pyramidal symptoms and signs can indeed be caused by risperidone on occasions. Sometimes extra pyramidal side effects can manifest with swallowing difficulties. Dr Jagus has reviewed your mother's case notes. Generally, it appears that she had been eating well and swallowing was not considered a problem throughout her admission. The first mention that there seemed to be a problem with actual eating was on the day of her admission to Noble's Hospital on 20 July 2012, where it was noticed that she was not chewing her sandwich, due to what was thought to be drowsiness, but she drank a glass of juice. There is no record of any problems with swallowing at this stage. The onset of altered conscious levels due to the presence of her infection at this stage is clearly influencing her ability to eat and this is noted. (Not in report. Nurse Halsall, on the first medical admission noted in written records that Judith had difficulty in swallowing, proving the above to be untrue).

Paragraph 2
Your mother was diagnosed with pyelonephritis which is a more severe form of a urinary tract infection, which had obviously caused a significant systemic infection and delirium. She went on to develop cholecystitis with infection of the gall bladder and bile duct, which again required intravenous antibiotics so was therefore seen as a more serious infection. However, as stated above, the mortality rate in delirium is very high irrespective of the speed at which the condition is treated.

Paragraph 3
We note that you believe her (report error), mother's dementia was in the early stages although accompanied by aggression and severe behavioural problems. The Psychiatric Team caring for your mother are of the opinion that her dementia was in the advanced stages. She was first seen in the memory clinic in 2008, and there had already been onset of worrying symptoms at this stage suggesting the condition probably started maybe 1-2 years before this in 2006 or 2007.

The average life expectancy of someone with Alzheimer's disease is 7 years in the absence of any major complications and so she was already approximately 4-5 years into this period. We have identified that in April 2011 your mother was tested using the Mini Mental State Examination (MMSE), which is a very widely recognised cognitive assessment. At this point she scored 12/30. The MMSE is recognised as a guide to the staging of Alzheimer's disease. Indeed, the recent NICE guidelines on dementia stated that Mild Dementia generally scored above 20/30, moderate was 16-20/30 and severe dementia was below 10/30. With a score of 12, she was clearly in the moderate to severe stage even in April 2011. The condition continued to progress after this, so we are of the opinion that she was clearly in the severe stages of illness during her lengthy admissions.

Paragraph 4
This refers to swelling of the face and neck – we hope that we have been able to address this earlier.

Paragraph 6

Dr Nordgard noted when he reviewed your mother on 20 July 2012 that her temperature was marginally raised at 37.5 degree Celsius. **(Not in the report, but very significant, on 20 July 2012, Judith's temperature was noted in Mental Health Records as 38.5 degrees).**

When you mother was admitted to the Surgical Ward at Noble's Hospital her temperature was 37.4 degrees. She then remained apyrexia (no temperature) until the early hours of 22 July 2012 when her temperature was recorded as being 37.8degrees. This was at 0150 hours. At 0345 hours her temperature was 37.5 degrees and by 0845 hours her temperature had come down to 35.6 degrees.

At 1435 hours on 27 July 2012 your mother's temperature was noted to be 37.5 degrees and when your mother returned to Grianagh Court her temperature was noted to be 37.3 degrees. This is just before being transferred back to Noble's Hospital with cholecystitis.

On your mother's readmission to the Medical Ward at Noble's Hospital, she was noted to have an increased temperature (i.e. higher than 37.5 degrees which would have triggered a score on the Noble's Warning Score System), on the following date-

28 July 2012	2100 hours	37.8 degrees Celsius
29 July 2012	1800 hours	37.5 degrees Celsius
31 July 2012	1855 hours	37.6 degrees Celsius
01 August 2012	0600 hours	37.9 degrees Celsius
01 August 2012	2150 hours	37.5 degrees Celsius
06 August 2012	1215 hours	37.6 degrees Celsius
06 August 2012	1310 hours	37.5 degrees Celsius
06 August 2012	1830 hours	37.5 degrees Celsius
09 August 2012	0725 hours	37.7 degrees Celsius
12 August 2012	1820 hours	37.6 degrees Celsius
26 August 2012	1815 hours	37.6 degrees Celsius

Paragraph 6

Please accept our apologies for the error. Your mother's medication chart has been reviewed and we can confirm that Nitrofurantoin 50 mgs 4 times a day was prescribed. (not 250mg 4 times, as detailed in Dr Jagus' report to the hospital), and this is within the recognised dosage range.

Paragraph 7

Dr Jagus prescribed Pregablin on 24 August 2011 when he reviewed your mother in his clinic at Mount View House, Ramsey. This was commenced in response to problems that both she and her husband reported about sleep disturbances, irritability, hostility, anxiety and a significant constant headache. Your father was finding managing your mother very difficult at this point and Dr Jagus and your father discussed various treatment options available. Pregablin is licensed for the treatment of generalised anxiety disorder and as such can have positive effects on irritability. As it can also be used for pain, it was felt that this may therefore be an appropriate treatment at this point based also on the presence of severe headaches. Dr Jagus was very aware that your mother was taking other sedative drugs so significant caution was used in the dosage of Pregablin. When it was commenced it was commenced at 25 mgs twice a day and based on the fact that the recommended minimum dose is 150 mgs a day, we hope that we have been able to reassure you that this is a very small dose. In terms of the reason the medication had been prescribed for your mother, it is because her dementia was characterised by high levels of personal distress and these treatments were used to at least give her some chance of peace and in an attempt to improve her day to day quality of life.

There has been no intention at any stage to deliberately overmedicate her. Pregablin was increased to 50 mgs 3 times a day on 10 February 2012 because again of significant concerns at Glen House around aggression, agitation and anxiety. However, 50 mgs three times a day is still only the minimum dose of Pregablin whose dosage is recommended up to 600mgs per day. (Not in report. This is not the recommended dose for elderly dementia patients, with interactions with Mirtazapine, Diazepam and Lorazepam noted in BNF).

Paragraph 8
The side effects of Nitrofurantoin have been looked in to as had various literature and we have been unable to locate any links between the use of medications and creatine kinase levels. We note that the bacterial culture result of your mother's urine sample taken on 12 July 2012 confirmed E-coli infection which was sensitive to Nitrofurantoin. This was the treatment of choice at that time as the organisms were resistant to the commonly used antibacterial agents.

Paragraph 9
Liver impairment can indeed impair the hepatic metabolism of Risperidone and the recommendations are that the doses are kept low or reduced rather than in being contraindication. As always in the cases, particularly in elderly patients, the dose of neuroleptics is always kept low. Indeed, when it was first commenced on 01 April 2012, the dose was only 0.5 mgs twice a day. Although your mother's liver function tests had been deranged for some time, the levels of AST, ALT, Bilirubin and GGT were relatively mildly elevated at various times and would not be indicative of significant hepatic impairment.

Paragraph 10
As we have previously explained, Dr Jagus did not visit your mother at Noble's Hospital until 31 July 2012. He had returned from annual leave on 23 July 2012 to be informed that your mother had been transferred to the hospital and was being treated for Pyelonephritis with intravenous antibiotics. In terms of clinical responsibility, as we have explained in a previous paragraph, at that point her clinical care and responsibility would have rested with the consultant in charge of her care at Noble's Hospital (Mr Mownah and then Dr Krishnan) and it would not necessarily have been appropriate for Dr Jagus to have reviewed her at this stage.

Your mother was undergoing acute treatment for severe infection at this stage and it was felt appropriate to allow them to treat her for this before reviewing her. Dr Jagus did call to review your mother on 31 July 2012 after she had returned back to Noble's Hospital following a period back at Grianagh Court when she was then thought to have cholecystitis which again was being treated was intravenous antibiotic. Dr Jagus was not asked to review her at this stage but felt it would be appropriate to monitor the situation. (This is untrue, as medics requested psychiatric reviews on 21 July and 30 July).

Conversely, if a patient is transferred from a medical ward to the care of a psychiatrist in Grianagh Court, it would not be appropriate for a Consultant from Noble's to review them unless requested.

Paragraph 11

Mrs Fell, Senior Practitioner had discussed your concern regarding a meeting that was never arranged. R.N. Dela Rosa recalls contacting you but is unfortunately unable to recall the exact details of how she followed this up. Dr Jagus met with you at Noble's Hospital on 07 September 2012. Mrs Fell recalls receiving an e-mail from you on 28 September 2012 in which you requested a meeting with Dr Jagus, as you still had concerns over your mother's care and Mrs Fell advised via e-mail on 02 October 2012, that a meeting had been arranged for 09 October 2012 at 1030 hours. You advised Mrs Fell again by e-mail on 04 October 2012 that you wished to cancel the meeting, as you believed that this was not the most appropriate channel to follow.

Paragraph 12

Your mother did become incapacitated when she was in Grianagh Court, but this was considered to be due to delirium due to significant infection which required her admission to Noble's Hospital, rather than as a result of medications.

Paragraph 13

We have always agreed that caution is required when prescribing sedative drugs and it is also correct that your mother was on combinations of potential sedative drugs at various stages. Please may we assure you that the staff were and are aware of combinations of sedative drugs that can have interactions. Consideration was made in dosages which can be very low or below the normal dosage range recommended in BNF for the medications. There were occasions where staff reviewed her medication, reduced the numbers and combination of psychotropic medications prescribed.

For example, on 11 June 2012 Dr Jagus was concerned that your mother had been on a number of psychotropic drugs with little overall effect on her levels of distress and agitation and so at that point the risperidone and pregabalin was reduced and her nightly sedation she had been taking at that point was stopped. The risperidone itself was stopped by Dr Jagus on 18 June 2012.

All the team involved in your mother's case say it is one of the more distressing cases of Alzheimer's disease they have treated. It was from the outset characterised by depression, agitation, high levels of distress and also psychotic symptoms in the form of hallucinations and delusional ideas often surrounding her husband. Much of the staff's attempts to treat this were around trying to give her some peace of mind and reduce her levels of distress and aggression.

We do sincerely extend our condolences to you and your family. We do hope that this response will help to answer your outstanding queries. Dr Jagus however, does feel that it would be appropriate to meet with you once more if you feel that this would help.

If having read our response, you feel a meeting would not be beneficial to clarify any residual issues arising out of your complaint, please do not hesitate to contact Amanda Mills".

Later that week Judith's medical records were eventually delivered, and evident missing records from the Mental Health were sent after further requesting them too.

Most notable events deduced from the Mental Health Records are observed as:-

12 July 2012 at Grianagh Court. Nursing staff noted increased urinary frequency/urgency and dark cloudy urine. Urine sample heavily positive for nitrates and leukocytes. Previous (20/6/12) MSU positive for multi-resistant E. Coli ESBC, which patient is now colonised with -Nitrofurantoin 50mgs QDS (4 x daily).

Lynne Merriman noted – spoke with infection control re multi resistant E.coli/ESBL. They stated no particular concern is needed – usual precaution e.g. gloves/apron (PPE) ordinary detergents used, no need for Chlorclean. ESBL is spread mostly by hands so excellent hand hygiene for staff and for Judith is necessary.

14 July 2012. Delia Dela Rosa noted Judith still restless and agitated. She appears angry, banging the main door and making fist towards staff. Contact Dr O'Sullivan and informed about Judith's behaviour this morning and this afternoon. She ordered 0.5mg risperidone and increased her diazepam to 15mg/24hrs.

Later on that day, Dr Marie O'Sullivan noted, plan – add Risperidone 0.5mgs bd to present meds.

16 July 2012, Dr Marie O'Sullivan noted, Judith has become more disturbed, with visual hallucinations and aggression toward residents, visitors and staff. Plan – to commence risperidone and gradually increase dose depending on response.

18 July 2012 05:20 hours; Delia Dela Rosa noted, Judith sat in the lounge at the end of the corridor, talking to herself. Observed leaning forward. (This "leaning forward", was notable enough to document. Presumably not "normal" leaning forward).

11:35 hours Sylvia McClafferty noted. Judith had a little sleep this morning. She is slightly unsteady on her feet and appears a little drowsy, though this has not stopped her from her usual walking up and down the corridor.

19:13 hours Margaret Halsall noted. Judith's mobility is poor today. Very stooped when walking, unsteady on her feet. Complaining of back pain.

19 July 2012 05:15 hours. John McKeefry noted. Incontinent of urine in bed, initially mobility was poor, but this has improved as the morning passed. Reviewed by Dr O'Sullivan who reduced risperidone to previous levels. Noted to have a tremor when trying to drink. F2 contacted and Procyclidine PRN written up.

19:17 hours. Delia Dela Rosa noted, observed not chewing her sandwich due to drowsiness, but consumed a glass of juice. Placed comfortably in small lounge and slept. Visited by her husband and was informed about Judith's condition and rashes on both legs.

20 July 2012 15:16 hours. Dr Kjell-Arne Norgard noted. Asked to see patient due to being drowsy and newly developed rashes on legs. Temp. 37.4 BP 140/70 HR 90 regular. Patient very somnolent and drowsy. When transferred to her room needed assistance from two staff when transferring to bed. Not responding adequately but opens eyes when being examined. O/E Dry tongue and mucous membranes. No signs of lymphadenopathy (glands that usually enlarge in response to a bacterial or viral infection), or icterus (jaundice) or anaemia. No leg swelling but newly developed papular rash on shins bilaterally. Heart sounds regular and clear. Lungs seem clear on auscultation and percussion, but poor air intake due to lack of compliance. Abdomen soft, bowel sounds present and seems tender in left flank. Imp:? Fever of unknown origin and dehydration. Maybe pyelonephritis (currently on Nitrofurantoin for UTI).

Plan: Bloods taken. CXR form filled out. Awaiting blood results before deciding if to call medical or surgical on call. Patient may need I.V. fluids since she is unable to drink.

(It was later this day, that R.N Halsall noted swelling in Judith's neck and her inability to swallow, as detailed in hospital letter. I was in attendance at this point and highlighted this too).

16:24 hours, Dr Nordgard noted; referred ptn to surgical SHO on call Dr Joshi, who kindly accepted the ptn to Ward 1. Nursing staff informed.

17.00 hours. R.N. Halsall noted. Phone call to Judith's husband informing him of transfer to Ward 1. Daughter visited information given re transfer. BP 150/75 **temp 38.5**

21 July 2012 09:52 hours. R.N. Halsall noted: Phone call from Ward 1 requesting review of Judith's Psychiatric medication. (incidentally this was done by Dr Slater and all medications were continued).

12:46 hours. Steward Slater noted. Reviewing regarding psychiatric medication on Ward 1 after discussion on G.C ward. Currently having Gentamycin and this to continue for further 24 hours. Judith seen to be taking small amounts of fluid orally and also her psychiatric medication. However, at present Judith lying quietly on bed when not asleep. This is attributed to tiredness, due to physical illness, where medics judge is **lower UTI rather than pyelonephritis.**

Plan: Pregablin reduced from 25 mgs tds to 25 mgs bd with view to stopping in 3 days. Instructions to omit diazepam doses if no indication that necessary. Ward 1 advised that we will take Judith back when medical intervention completed.

22 July 2012 10:58 hours. Bill Burnie noted. Seen on Ward 1, settled evening remains drowsy or asleep most of the time.

(The evening of 27 July 2012, Judith was returned to Grianagh Court. This was two days later than expected, as Grianagh Court did not have a free bed for Judith).

28 July 2012 05:18 hours, Natasha Moore noted: Judith in bed on commencement of shift, appeared sleepy although responsive. Staff tried to give Judith a drink, however **she had difficulty swallowing same. Mouth very dry and neck appears swollen.**

Unknown time or author but would appear to be Psychiatric Consultant.

Treated at Noble's **for queried pyelonephritis, which was ruled out**, as reported by Dr Joshi. Currently query treatment, resistant uti, sepsis.

On review decreased psychomotor drive, very limited verbal contact, does not accept food or fluids. Referral to Ward 6 discussed and agreed with Dr Noor.

Notes: **Procyclidine was prescribed on 19 July 2012, for "extra**

pyramidal symptom". That was a noticeable tremor when attempting to drink.

Notes End.

The list of medications that were prescribed at the time, were-

Mirtazapine	three x daily
Sodium Valproate	100mgs three x daily
Donezepil	10mgs once daily
Furosemide	**20 mg** /45mgs at night (Why is furosemide being prescribed at night?)
Diazepam	5mgs three x daily
Pregablin	25mgs **x twice daily**
Risperidone	**0.5 mgs twice daily**
Lanzoprazole	30 mgs once daily
Mebeverine	135mgs once daily
Procyclidine	2.5mg up to three x daily

Janssen-Cilag Ltd, the manufacturers of Risperdal – risperidone, (a subsidiary company of Johnson & Johnson), in their Patient Leaflet (www.medicines.org.uk/emc/product/6856/smpc) details-

Elderly patients with dementia.

Increased mortality in elderly people with dementia

There is a further increased risk of mortality in elderly dementia patients when Furosemide and Risperidone are concomitantly prescribed.

(For clarification purposes, Risperidone was commenced for the second time (since 19 June 2012), on 14 July 2012 at 0.5 mgs twice daily. On 16 July 2012 it was increased to 1 mg twice daily. On 19 July 2012 it was reduced back to 0.5mgs. The reason for the reduction in this must have been solely due to Judith's deterioration in physical capacity and presentation. Risperidone was being co-prescribed with Furosemide too).

The UK NHS provides information on Neuroleptic Malignant Syndrome, prepared by UK Medicines Information (UKMI), pharmacists for NHS Healthcare professionals.

They note:-

The majority of cases are caused by antipsychotic medication, but other drugs with dopaminergic action may also be implicated.

Symptoms

Onset is abrupt and symptoms progress rapidly over 24-72 hours. Following withdrawal of the causative drug, most patients recover with within 7 to 10 days, and virtually all patients recover within 30 days, but symptoms may be prolonged when long-acting depot injections are implicated. A significant minority of patients may suffer **long-term sequelae**, including neurological impairment, muscle contraction and cognitive deficits.

(*Bold indicates symptoms that Judith presented with*).

<u>Groups of symptoms and signs of Neuroleptic Malignant Syndrome</u>

Drowsiness, Confusion, Stupor, Coma
Delirium
Grand mal seizures
Hyperthermia (temperature over 38.5 degrees Celsius)
Autonomic instability
Tachycardia (rapid heartbeat)
Diaphoresis (sweating)
Incontinence
Tachypnoea (fast shallow breathing)
High arterial blood pressure
Muscle rigidity
Creatine Kinase markedly raised
Extra pyramidal symptoms
Trismus (jaw contraction)

Lead pipe rigidity
Rhabdomyolysis
Opisthotonus (state of severe hyperextension and spasticity in which an individual's head, neck and spinal column enter into a complete bridging or arching position).
Babinski's sign (abnormal flexion of the toes).
Chorea (abnormal involuntary movement disorder)
Laboratory Findings
Creatine Kinase is markedly increased.
Leukocytosis is present in up to 75% of cases.
Impaired liver function tests.
ECG abnormalities and electrolyte disturbances may also be present.
Cerebral CT scans and lumbar puncture are usually normal.

Summary

Neuroleptic Malignant Syndrome is a rare but serious idiosyncratic drug reaction.

An awareness of the risk factors, causative agents and symptoms is essential as NMS is a potentially fatal condition.

Early recognition of the syndrome may improve management and decrease mortality, so clinicians should be aware of which drugs can cause NMS and how diagnosis is made.

Neuroleptic Malignant Syndrome Clinical Presentation (http;// emedicine,medscape.com/article/242-clinical. Author J Tonkology et al), summarises features to be:-

Diaphoresis (sweating), **Dysphasia** (difficulty swallowing), **tremor**, **incontinence**, **delirium progressing to lethargy, stupor and coma**; **pallor**, dyspnea, **psychomotor agitation, rigidity**, **hyperthermia**, tachycardia, **shuffling gait**. Other features include a **rash**.

A most interesting publication is, "Catatonia in Medically Ill Patients, Evidence based Medicine (EMB) Monograph for Psychosomatic Medicine Practice", published jointly by The Guidelines and Evidence-Based Medicine Subcommittee of the Academy of Psychosomatic Medicine (APM) and the European Association of Psychosomatic Medicine (EAPM). Authors L Denysenko et al.

This report explains different types of catatonia and the many features and symptoms.

My main area of focus is on the section entitled, "Malignant Catatonia":-

"Malignant Catatonia is characterised by severe catatonia with muscle rigidity, hyperthermia, autonomic nervous system instability, delirium and agitation, which can then proceed to coma and death. It has also been called lethal catatonia.

When malignant catatonia occurs in the setting of exposure to dopamine antagonists (most antipsychotics, including risperidone), it has been called Neuroleptic Malignant Syndrome (NMS). Both disorders share many signs and symptoms. However, the term is misleading because NMS also can occur after abrupt discontinuation of dopamine antagonists, and after exposure to agents that are not considered dopamine antagonists. The DSM-5 (The Diagnostic and Statistical Manual of Mental Disorders, fifth edition), recognises that malignant catatonia may be indistinguishable from NMS. For the purpose of this monograph malignant catatonia and NMS are viewed as the same condition.

Definition and Diagnostic Criteria.

Catatonia is a neuropsychiatry syndrome with motor, vocal, affective, and behavioural peculiarities, including alterations in external and internal awareness. Features may include mutism or impoverished/ quiet speech, reduced interaction with the environment (stupor), negativism, increased motor tone/rigidity, posturing and grimacing, (this is not exhaustive of the extract).

There does not appear to be any evidence in the literature that validates the exclusion of catatonia as a diagnosis in patients with delirium. Furthermore, in NMS delirium is recognised as a diagnostic feature.

In conclusion, malignant catatonia has gone by many different names. A lack of open communication between medical disciplines has further compounded the problem, with different fields ascribing their own name or multiple names to the same syndrome. While further research is needed to better characterize malignant catatonia in its various forms, the medical community should also work on a unified model for better conceptualization of this syndrome.

The glossary of terms includes:-

Negativism:- an observable sign as well as a physical examination find, usually in catatonia but also in other conditions, including autism spectrum disorder, intellectual disability and traumatic brain injury. It is a phenomenon in which the patient refuses or does the opposite of what is asked or physically attempted by the examiner, in a manner that appears detached from a clearly identifiable motive. Motoric negativism can progress to negativity. **Refusal to eat or drink may also be viewed as a form of negativism**. Negativism is often misinterpreted as volitional uncooperativeness.

Posturing:- an observable sign in catatonia, in which the patient spontaneously develops and maintains a rigid, immobile posture, and maintains the posture for an abnormally long period of time. The posture may appear exaggerated, grotesque, bizarre and contorting, or it may appear superficially ordinary and underwhelming, such as sitting in a chair or bed abnormally still and with a tense appearance. Psychological pillow is a form of posturing in which a supine patient spontaneously develops and maintains a head posture above the plane of the bed without apparent effort or strain".

27

Assumptions and Presumptions

Another aspect of dementia that I was to learn is that Alzheimer's disease is the most common type of dementia, but the second/third, (depending on literature), most common dementia is Lewy Bodies Dementia (LBD).

The Central Feature of LBD is progressive dementia – deficits in attention and executive function are typical. Prominent memory impairment may not be evident in the early stages.

The Core Features of LBD is fluctuating with pronounced variations in attention and alertness. Recurrent complex visual hallucinations, typically well-formed and detailed.

Spontaneous features of Parkinsonism.

Suggested Features are-

Severe sensitivity to neuroleptics occur in up to 50% of LBD patients who take them.

Low dopamine transporter uptake in the brain's basal ganglia, as seen on SPECT and PET imaging scans.

Supportive Features;-

Repeated fall and fainting

Transient, unexplained loss of consciousness.

Autonomic dysfunction.

Hallucination of other senses, like touch and hearing.
Visuospatial abnormalities.
Other psychiatric disturbances.
(Above extract taken from Lewy Body Dementia Association, Inc).

I had no idea that Alzheimer's and Lewy Body Dementia were so similar, and it is likely that most patients will get diagnosed with Alzheimer's Disease, based on the concept that Alzheimer's is the most common dementia. A high-profile death through Lewy Body Dementia was actor, Robin Williams. It was upon autopsy, that a coroner found signs of LBD, and doctors who analysed the autopsy report told his wife, Susan, that it was one of the most severe cases they had ever seen. After his death, the Lewy Body Dementia Association detailed, "It takes an average of three doctors and more than 18 months to correctly diagnose LBD. Most doctors fail to recognise the signs of LBD; the symptoms are very similar to Alzheimer's disease and other neurodegenerative disorders, such as Parkinson's Disease".

Based on the one simple fact that up to 50% of the LBD patients will be severely sensitive to neuroleptic medication, I find this very, very, disturbing indeed. It is like playing "Russian Roulette" with a person's life. It is deeply concerning.

Reckless prescribing of psychiatric medication, coupled with the dangers of polypharmacy, and up to a 50% chance of developing Neuroleptic Malignant Syndrome if subjected to antipsychotic medication, seems quite astounding. Common sense must prevail and more needs to be done to protect this vulnerable population of elderly, dementia patients.

In the meantime, my father remained in the Rehabilitation ward for months. His mobility was not good and he had daily physiotherapy to improve his walking. Gradually he began to be able to eat and drink independently, but he was very frail.

Correspondence between myself and the hospital continued for well-over one year. I noted in Judith's medical records that when her Consultant Psychiatrist had input into the medical notes at the hospital, that he wrote "advanced dementia", in direct conflict to the "early stages, be it rapidly progressing", that he had explained to us, just over one month prior to Judith's death.

When the "Local Resolution" with the hospital had been exhausted and my questions were being ignored completely, I continued with the Independent Review Body complaints procedure. Although I do think that, "Independent" is extremely misleading.

Between these two processes I had contacted an Isle of Man politician, Kate Beecroft, at the forefront of concerns regarding the standards at the hospital. She put me in contact with a doctor, Dr Hulme, who regularly visited the island, and who had property on the island that used to be her late-mother's, in Peel. I was invited by her to the magnificent property overlooking Peel bay, and she requested that I brought my mother's medical records for her to peruse over a couple of days. She was shocked after reading them, and explained that doctors had misled me, especially when informing me that my mother was not dehydrated on admission to Noble's Hospital. She contacted her "business partner" who was in a pharmaceutical position to look at the combined medication that my mother had been taking. He informed her that the combination of drugs would have, "sedated an elephant". She informed me that the medics at Noble's Hospital clearly had no idea as to what was causing my mother's condition. She explained that my mother certainly did not have a kidney infection on her first admission to Noble's; her recorded temperatures alone were not elevated enough to indicate this. Dr Hulme had been a G.P. for most of her working life in Shifnal in Staffordshire. She also suggested that I report Dr Jagus to the GMC, but I had already done this. The GMC dismissed my concerns as "a hospital issue" and suggested that I also contact the Independent Review Body on the Island, providing the contact details.

Sometime later, I received the letter, detailing the arrangements for the Independent Review Body meeting:-

"Dear Mrs Quine

Further to recent correspondence, I am pleased to confirm the Hearing will take place on Wednesday 1 October 2014 at the Manx Blind Welfare Society Building in Onchan and it is anticipated that your attendance will be requested in the morning. You are entitled to be accompanied by a friend, who may also speak on your behalf, but cannot be represented by a legal representative acting as such.

The Terms of Reference are contained in the indented list below. Should you wish to make any comment on these, you are required to do so in writing within 10 working days of the date of this letter.

To consider whether the treatment and medication regime being offered to Mrs Allen at Grianagh Court from April 2012 to her Admission to Noble's Hospital on 20 July 2012 (with particular reference to the combination of medications, and the treatment of delirium), was of a standard which could reasonably be expected.

To consider whether other health care professionals in similar circumstances would have considered Mrs Allen to be suffering from Neuroleptic Malignant Syndrome.

To consider whether staff at Noble's Hospital were given sufficient information on Mrs Allen's various conditions, (including delirium) when she was admitted in July 2012, to enable her to be treated appropriately.

A venue location map will be available nearer the date together with full details of attendees and timings. In this connection, it would be helpful for me to meet with you before the date of the hearing to explain the arrangements and procedure, please let me know.

Yours sincerely
Andrea Roberts
Clerk, Independent Review Body"

Following the receipt of the letter, I replied on 2 June 2014:

"Thank you for your recent letter dated 20 June 20014, informing me of the Hearing taking place on Wednesday, 01 October 2014. I confirm that I will be in attendance of this.

With regards to the terms of reference, I have the following comments to make:

With regards to polypharmacy, this must have put Judith at particularly high risk of likely adverse reactions, especially given the concomitant use of Risperidone and Furosemide. The clear risk of dehydration added even further to the high risk of mortality. I would also like to question what scans were undertaken to determine the type of dementia, prior to the prescribing of Risperidone and what the norms would be.

Are health care professionals here trained to recognise symptoms of NMS? Have any been reported on the Isle of Man? I note that she was given Procyclidine for extra pyramidal symptoms, just one day prior to her hospital admission.

The death certificate must be factually incorrect. Hospital staff even noted the patient singing along to a C.D. just over one week prior to her death. I have a voice recording of her answering questions too. Surely this is not consistent with last stage dementia behaviour.

Most importantly, I am concerned that it was imperative that the medications, and in particular Risperidone, should have been stopped. Yet the two doctors made, what I believe to be a fully informed decision to mislead us and inform us that in meetings, (with others present, and that are voice recorded), that the medication was firstly not taken during the hospital admission, and then that it had been stopped, and therefore not taken.

As part of the Hospital Complaints process, the hospital report itself confirms that the medication was indeed still taken upon admission, and for a considerable time after -nearly eleven days.

At what point should the hospital have taken these deliberate cover-ups seriously, and have taken serious action?

A worryingly dangerous complaint was already in place, two months prior to the death, made by our family. Yet despite cover-ups being made, the hospital continued to gloss-over the fact that two doctors felt the need to lie. This really must be an offence.

These are just some of the points that I would like raising during the hearing if possible.

I would also very much like to obtain further details with regards to the procedures and arrangements, along with the details of who will be attending too".

In reply to my letter, I received a detailed outline of the hearing;-

"Date: 01 October 2014
Time: From 9.30am
Venue: Manx Blind Welfare Headquarters
Panel Members:
Mr A Guy {Chairman}
Mrs V Hare {Convenor}
Mr C Brown {Lay member}
Mrs A Roberts {IRB Clerk} in attendance

Assessors:
Mrs D Cope, Associate Medical Director/Lead for Revalidation
Mr L Mynors-Wallis, Medical Director/Consultant Psychiatrist
Ms C Young, Practice Development Nurse, End of Life Care

Approximate schedule for hearing:
9.30am. Mrs Victoria Quine and Sophie Allen
11am Dr C Jagus, Consultant Psychiatrist, Older Persons' Mental Health Service, to be accompanied by Mrs S Waddecar, Patient Safety and Quality Office, Noble's Hospital.
2.00pm Dr Balakrishnan, Consultant Physician, Noble's Hospital.
3.00pm Mrs B Scott, Hospital Manager, Noble's Hospital

3.45pm Dr T Byrne, Clinical Director, Mental Health, Noble's Hospital.

The panel will sit in private at the conclusion of the Hearing, which is expected to be from approximately 4.30pm.

Terms of reference-

To consider whether the treatment and medication regime being offered to Mrs Allen at Grianagh Court from April 2012 to her admission to Noble's 20 July 2012 with particular reference to the combination of medications, and the treatment of delirium, was of a standard which could be reasonably expected.

To consider whether other healthcare professionals in similar circumstances would have considered Mrs Allen to be suffering from Neuroleptic Malignant Syndrome.

To consider whether Staff at Noble's Hospital were given sufficient information on Mrs Allen's conditions, including delirium, when she was admitted in July 2012, to enable her to be treated appropriately.

To consider whether Mrs Allen was appropriately placed on the Liverpool Care Pathway." End.

Not long after receiving the Hearing details, Andrea Roberts from the Independent Review Body came to my house. We had sat in the lounge discussing the events surrounding my mother's death, and the procedure for the Hearing. I then compiled, at her request, a list of questions that she would put forward to the professional doctors who would visit the island from the UK and who would investigate my complaint regarding Judith's death and treatment.

In the meantime, Kate Beecroft had introduced me to a couple of people who had similar personal experiences with the hospital and who had been through the Independent Review Body Complaints process. Both individuals had inferred that the procedure was really more of a damage limitation exercise, as opposed to a "Hearing", as the I.R.B. referred to it. I liked to consider myself as open-minded and with two top, professionally recognised doctors in their field of expertise, I hoped that this would not be a "paid for consultation". I had hoped for a Pharmacologist, or a Physician to be on the Assessors panel, as opposed to two psychiatrists, who worked at the same NHS Hospital, in similar positions, with almost the same areas of expertise too. One of whom, Dr Mynors-Wallis, was a medico-legal consultant also.

The night prior to the meeting, I felt very anxious. It had taken nearly two years to get to this point. I really needed some answers to my very relevant questions. I felt reassured that Andrea Roberts had my list of questions and points to be raised, that she had written out whilst visiting me at home.

Early in the morning, Sophie drove over the mountain road from Ramsey. She was still unaware of the full extent of the lack of care, and horrendous experiences that her grandmother had suffered. I didn't want to add to the grieving that she was still going through. My parents had regularly child-minded Sophie throughout her childhood and she had therefore been close to them. I hoped the meeting wouldn't prove too traumatic for her. I prayed for my composure too.

I was so nervous driving up to the meeting. It felt like attending the biggest, most important job interview. I knew I wasn't articulate or confident under such circumstances, but I just wished for my honesty to be enough to help me through.

Now, at this point, I knew that I wouldn't be allowed to record the meeting; from people who had experienced the IRB Hearing for themselves, and the simple fact that no legal representation was allowed either. Recording would be a certain "no no". Yet, despite this, I knew that for the safety of other people who might be subjected to such treatment, I needed to remember the sequence of events and how complainants were being treated, especially with the lack of confidence in the hospital standards that was surrounding it. Therefore, in the car when I parked up, I set my iPad to record, before we entered into the building.

Sophie and I arrived and sat in the foyer of the building. Andrea Roberts came to great us and explained that she would call us when the members were ready for us. Mrs Hare and Mr Guy questioned me to ensure I understood the process was "Independent".

Once inside, I sifted through my handbag, setting my purse and my iPad on the table in front of me, while I retrieved my pen, to appear to be taking notes. I had learned by now, and with good reason, to trust nobody. Sadly, it was only our meeting that morning that could be recorded though.

Inside the meeting room, we sat around a huge table. It seemed too big and a little intimidating, but thankfully the distance between the attendees was beneficial for recording purposes. Everybody appeared very chilled and relaxed apart from me. I was shaking but trying my hardest to remain calm. I remembered to bring water, that would stave-off my terribly dry mouth when under pressure, but at that point I could not lift the bottle as I was trembling too much. During the meeting my honesty would be pure and unadulterated; of that I was proud. Sophie and I sat next to each other. All eyes were on us.

Introductions were formally made. Then we commenced to discuss the start of my mother's dementia and the course of events, leading up to her first assessment in Grianagh Court.

Dr Mynors-Wallis asked if my mother was calmer when we visited her. We explained that she was and would often run to the door to greet my father, and always recognised family members. Sometimes she would introduce me as her sister to people, but she never failed to recognise us and hug us. The word, "sister", may have been a mix-up on her words, but the recognition was always there. Both myself and Sophie explained that Judith was suffering with hallucinations for some considerable time; talking to imaginary children and animals.

We explained that her appetite was very good prior to her admission to Noble's Hospital.

I informed him of the events prior to her hospital admission, highlighting the bizarre posture that she had on 19 July, just one day before the admission from Grianagh Court to Noble's Hospital. I told the hearing how she was sitting in an impossible posture, unable to move, or talk or drink. (I physically demonstrated the posture to the IRB attendees).

I went on to explain that as a child, I had suffered an oculogyric crisis, where my neck was bents backwards and my eyes were rolled into my head too, which was the result of an adverse drug reaction to medication that I had taken. I provided Dr Mynors-Wallis with a print-out of this from my doctor's surgery, reiterating why, in my opinion, I considered Judith was having an adverse reaction to medication.

I detailed to the hearing, the swelling that was in my mother's neck, forearms and face, and explained that unlike normal swelling, my fingers did not depress into my mother's skin; the swelling was solid. I informed them about how Judith had lost her mobility, talking and eating on the day prior to her first admission to Noble's hospital.

Sophie explained that on the day prior to Judith's death, she had read her grandmother a story and when Sophie finished reading, and asked her granny if she enjoyed it, Judith squeezed her hand and smiled. Judith then said that she didn't want to die.

I told the hearing that I had wished the hospital had taken our complaint seriously and wished they had put measures in place to ensure this never happened to another vulnerable dementia patient. I told of how the Sister on the ward, raised her concerns with me about the risperidone medication, and how she had written the drug name down for me, and how, further to research from the patient information leaflet, I was totally convinced that my mother had suffered from Neuroleptic Malignant Syndrome. It was my opinion that it was concurrent with a urinary tract infection too. All concerned at the hearing, admitted to reading Judith's notes, and also my correspondence with the hospital.

I confirmed that I thought Judith's incapacitation and demise was due to undetected Neuroleptic Malignant Syndrome. Sophie believed that her grandmother was suffering from anorexia and refused to eat. We both explained that Judith was too lucid to be in the last stages of dementia, in our opinion. We both agreed though, that Judith did have dementia.

For some unknown reason, Dr Mynors-Wallis, at the end of the meeting wished to take photocopies of the notes I had taken. I agreed to this, as I had nothing to hide.

We were both taken to sit in the foyer again, while the notes took an exceptionally long time to be photocopied. During this time, Dr Jagus arrived, but went straight to the washroom, and remained there until we had left. I had no wish to sit in his company.

28

Tainted Transparency

The report arrived in January 2015, nearly three months after the report date:-

Independent Review into the Complaint of Mrs Quine in Respect of Treatment Received by her Mother, the Late Judith Allen.

Dr Laurence Mynors-Wallis
Medical Director/Consultant Psychiatrist
Dorset Healthcare University NHS Foundation Trust

Dr Denise Cope
Associate Medical Director
Dorset Healthcare University NHS Foundation Trust

23 October 2014

First page is indexed of contents.

Introduction

1.1 This report has been prepared at the request of the Isle of Man Independent Review Body (IRB), to investigate the complaint of Mrs Quine, in respect of the treatment received by her late mother, Mrs Judith Allen.

1.2 In preparation of this report, Dr Mynors-Wallis and Dr Cope read eight volumes of medical records sent to us by the IRB. We also participated in a full day hearing on 01 October 2014, during which the following were interviewed:-

I) Mrs Victoria Quine accompanied by her daughter, Sophie Allen.
II) Dr C Jagus, Consultant Psychiatrist, Older Peoples Mental Health Service, Noble's Hospital.
III) Dr V Balakrishnan, Consultant Physician, Noble's Hospital.
IV) Mrs B Scott, Hospital Manager, Noble's Hospital.
V) Dr T Byrne, Clinical Director, Mental Health Services, Noble's Hospital.

1.3 Dr Cope and Dr Mynors-Wallis were appointed by the IRB to act as independent assessors in the review of the complaint.

1.4 Dr Mynors-Wallis is a Consultant Psychiatrist and the Medical Director of Dorset Healthcare University NHS Foundation Trust and a Visiting Professor at Bournemouth University. He qualified in medicine in 1984 and spent 18 months gaining experience in general medicine. He obtained his membership of the Royal College of Physicians in 1987. He did his initial training in psychiatry at the Maudsley Hospital in London, together with a six month attachment at the Royal Prince Albert Hospital in Sydney. He became a member of the Royal College of Psychiatrists in 1989, obtaining the Laughlin Prize for the best examination results in that year. He then obtained a Wellcome Trust Training Fellowship to study the treatment of depressive disorders in primary care, obtaining a Doctorate in Medicine from Oxford University in 1994. He has been a Consultant Psychiatrist since 1995. He has scientific publications in the field of depressive and emotional disorders. He was a foundation Council member of the Faculty of Medical Leadership and Management. He is the Registrar for the Royal College of Psychiatrists with lead responsibility for public information, policy and the revalidation of consultant psychiatrists. He has been trained to assess and supervise doctors who have restrictions on the registration, for the General Medical Council. He was awarded a Fellowship of the Royal College of Psychiatrists in 2008.

1.5 Dr Cope is a Consultant Old Age Psychiatrist and works as an Associate Medical Director at Dorset Healthcare University NHS Foundation Trust. She is responsible for administering the system for appraisal and the revalidation of doctors within this organisation. She is an Associate Postgraduate Dean with Health Education Wessex. She is Clinical Lead for Mental Health and Dementia in the Wessex Strategic Clinical Network, part of the NHS England. She qualified in medicine in 1982. Her initial postgraduate training was aimed at a career in general practice. She obtained her membership of the Royal College of General Practitioners in 1987. Her training in psychiatry began in 1986. The majority of her training occurred in Wessex region. She became a member of the Royal College of Psychiatrists in 1989. She was appointed to a Consultant post in Old Age Psychiatry in Dorset in 1991. She was awarded a Fellowship of the Royal College of Psychiatrists in 2002.

2. Terms of Reference.

2.1 The Terms of Reference for the hearing which we understand we agreed with Mrs Quine were as follows:-

I) To consider whether the treatment and medication regime being offered to Mrs Allen at Grianagh Court from April 2012 to her admission to Noble's Hospital on 20 July 2012 with particular reference to the combination of medications, (and the treatment of delirium), was of a standard which could reasonably be expected.

II) To consider whether other healthcare professionals in similar circumstance would have considered Mrs Allen to be suffering from Neuroleptic Malignant Syndrome.

III) To consider whether staff at Noble's Hospital were given sufficient information on Mrs Allen's various conditions (including delirium), when she was admitted in July 2012 to enable her to be treated appropriately.

IV) To consider whether Mrs Allen was appropriately placed on the Liverpool Care Pathway. This question will be answered by an appropriate specialist.

2.2 This report will consider only the first three questions. Question Four is being answered by another expert.

3. Outline of Mrs Allen's Relevant Medical History.

3.1 Mrs Allen was seen by specialist mental health services in 2011. Mrs Allen's husband had been admitted to hospital with a possible seizure; he had been providing significant care for his wife. Mrs Allen's family were concerned about her memory and behavioural problems, and her husband's ability to cope. Mrs Allen was assessed by Dr Jagus, Consultant Old Age Psychiatrist on 20 April 2011. A diagnosis of dementia was made. Mrs Allen and her husband were subsequently supported in the community by members of Dr Jagus' mental health team.

3.2 In October 2011, Mr Allen was admitted to hospital having had a stroke. Mrs Allen was being aggressive with family members, for example, trying to strangle them. She had poor short-term memory. At times she did not recognise family members; she would leave the house and go wandering and be brought back by neighbours. Mrs Allen needed help with self-care, including going to the toilet, washing, and dressing. She was anxious and tearful.

3.3 On 30 October 2011, Mrs Allen was admitted to Grianagh Court. On admission she was reported as tearful and incoherent and had difficulty in answering questions put to her. She was reported as being very anxious and agitated. She could not remember her age, date of birth and was unaware of where she was or what date it was. Mrs Quine informed us that she was aware that the purpose of the assessment was to assess her mother and then identify a suitable residential placement.

3.4 Mrs Allen was an inpatient in Grianagh Court until 25 November 2011, when she was admitted to the Glen House Residential Home. On 2 February 2012, Mrs Allen moved from Glen House to Beaconsfield Towers Nursing Home. The move was a result of the Glen House staff being unable to meet Mrs Allen's behaviour, in particular, her aggression towards staff and her increasing care needs. Staff at Beaconsfield Towers quickly came to the opinion that they were also unable to meet Mrs Allen's needs because of her aggressive behaviour and agitation.

3.5. On 02 April 2012, Mrs Allen was readmitted to Grianagh Court on Section 2 of the Mental Health Act. Mrs Allen continued to be irritable, distressed and tearful at times and would hit out at staff and fellow patients. She needed help with all self-care activities. She was reported to be disorientated, in person, place and time.

3.6 From reviewing of the RiO notes and available medication charts, it appears that the psychotropic medications used during this admission were as follows-

I) Donezepil – an anti-dementia drug
II) Memantine – an anti-dementia drug
III) Chloral Betaine – a hypnotic
IV) Mirtazapine – an antidepressant
V) Lorazepam – an anti-anxiety drug
VI) Diazepam – an anti-anxiety drug
VII) Pregablin – an anti-anxiety drug
VIII) Sodium Valproate – a mood stabiliser
IX) Risperidone – an antipsychotic

(Not in report. I specifically asked for the Furosemide script to be addressed. It never was).

3.7 No care plan for non-pharmacological interventions, consent issues or family involvement could be found in the case notes.

3.8 On 27 April 2012, it is recorded that although Mrs Allen remained disorientated, anxious and agitated, she was compliant with medication and care and was not making clear and persistent attempts to leave. Therefore, the Section 2 of the Mental Health Act was discharged.

3.9 During the second phase in Grianagh Court, it was recorded that Mrs Allen required assistance from up to three staff to wash and dress her. She became incontinent of urine and faeces. She remained emotionally very labile. Dr Jagus reported that Mrs Allen was very distressed at times.

3.10 During the days prior to Mrs Allen's transfer from Grianagh Court, her mental and physical state changed; her presentation fluctuated. She developed visual hallucinations, was variably agitated and distressed and at times had disturbed consciousness. She was lethargic being unable to take food and liquid consistently. This change coincided with the time she was presumed to be developing a urinary tract infection. The symptoms described in the notes of her presentation support a delirium diagnosis.

3.11 On 20 July 2012, Mrs Allen became drowsy and had a temperature. She was transferred to a medical ward at Noble's Hospital, where a diagnosis of pyelonephritis was made. Mrs Allen remained in the medical wards at Noble's until her death on 20 October 2012. (Error, should read 25 October).

3.12 Reviewing RiO mental health records there is little documentation about formal, regular communication with family members by the multi-professional team. Dr Jagus was clear with us at interview that he did have meetings with Mr Allen during outpatient assessments of his wife and during those shared information about diagnosis, prognosis and management.

4. OPINION:

Whether the treatment and medication being offered to Mrs Allen at Grianagh Court from April 2012 to her admission to Noble's on 20 July 2012 (with particular reference to the combination of medications and the treatment of delirium), was of a standard which could be reasonably expected.

4.1 During the period under consideration, Mrs Allen was an inpatient at Grianagh Court having been admitted from Beaconsfield Nursing Home. The admission occurred under Section 2 of the Mental Health Act. The reason for admission was increasing behaviours that challenged within the context of a moderate to severe dementia. Mrs Allen was transferred from Grianagh Court to Ward 1 at Noble's Hospital on 20 July 2012 due to deterioration of her physical health and a presumed urinary tract infection.

4.2 Mrs Allen's presenting symptoms requiring admission, assessment and management varied over time, but included anxiety, restlessness, agitation, resistive behaviours and most significant hostility and physical aggression to other patients, staff and occasional family members. These can be summarised as behavioural and psychological symptoms of dementia. Visual hallucinations and occasional auditory hallucinations are recorded within the case notes and appear to have fluctuated over time. These symptoms occur in moderate and severe dementia.

4.3 Use of medications for the symptoms presented by Mrs Allen should be considered after, or in combination with non-pharmacological interventions. During the interview with Dr Jagus, he stated that relaxation techniques, use of a sensory room, ward activities and use of quiet areas of the ward were the non-pharmacological interventions used in Grianagh Court. There is occasional reference within the notes to the use of 1:1 time, taking Mrs Allen into the garden on several occasions and a single reference to a sensory machine being used. There is no documented evidence of systematic use of non-pharmacological interventions or details of the content of 1:1 time and its effectiveness. It is our opinion that the failure to write up a care plan, setting out non-pharmacological interventions being used in Mrs Allen's care fell below best practice standards.

4.4 Our opinion on medication will be limited to the psychotropic medications prescribed during the admission to Grianagh Court and the appropriateness of their use to manage the behavioural and psychological symptoms listed in paragraph 3 above.

4.5 During the interview with Dr Jagus, he shared with us his rationale for medications used and explained that no formal monitoring of target symptoms occurred. He did state that clinical judgement of response to medications, guided prescribing decisions. Review of the RiO notes does not provide evidence of this being documented to support any changes in medication regime that occurred. It is our opinion that although many medical records will not contain the clear rationale for the changing medication and formal monitoring of target symptoms, this would be an area of good practice and we recommend that the medical team on the ward adopt the recommendations set out below to improve practice.

4.6 We will review each medication listed in paragraph 3 above, the licenses indications and the rationale for its use in the treatment of Mrs Allen, together with our opinion on the appropriateness of each medication used.

I) Donepezil Hydrochloride. The licensed indication for this medication is mild to moderate dementia in Alzheimer's Disease. This was an appropriate prescription for Mrs Allen during her admission to Grianagh Court. (Not in report. The Canadian Government withdrew Donepezil use, as they found can cause Neuroleptic Malignant Syndrome).

II) Memantine. The licensed indication for this medication is moderate to severe Alzheimer's Disease. This was an appropriate prescription for Mrs Allen. The medication was discontinued on 21 May 2012. The documented reason in Rio notes was that it can possibly cause agitation.

III) Chloral Betaine. The licensed indication for this medication in insomnia – short-term use. Mrs Allen was taking this medication prior to her admission to Grianagh Court. Dr Jagus informed us at interview that other night sedatives had been tried and failed to deal with what he described as severe insomnia. During Mrs Allen's admission to Grianagh Court, insomnia was not identified as a problem and the medication was stopped on 11 June 2012 with no adverse effect. Use of a night sedative beyond short-term use indication needs to be made carefully. This can be justified in a patient with dementing illness where the sleep pattern is particularly disturbed. The use of Chloral Betaine appeared to resolve Mrs Allen's sleeping problem. It is our opinion that the use of Chloral Betaine could be justified.

(Not in the report, but significant; Chloral Betaine had been prescribed to Judith for at least eight months).

IV) Mirtazapine. The licensed indication for this medication is major depression. Mrs Allen was admitted to Grianagh Court on this medication and had been a long-term treatment for depressive symptoms, which were diagnosed when she was initially assessed. Discussion with Dr Jagus indicated that the medication had had a beneficial effect and, in view of her on-going agitation and distress, a decision was made to continue this. It is our opinion that the use of Mirtazapine was appropriate.

(Not in report, but significant: Mirtazapine can cause the potentially fatal Neuroleptic Malignant Syndrome. Judith continued with this prescription during Noble's Hospital admission. It is known to cause agitation, aggression and confusion. This was one of Judith's longest standing medication; approximately four years, with no review).

V) Lorazepam and Diazepam. These two medications are benzodiazepines and are licensed for short-term use in anxiety or insomnia. In the situation presented by Mrs Allen both medications were used for acute short-term control of agitation and aggressive behaviour. It is our opinion that the use of these drugs in this context was justified.

VI) Pregablin. This medication is licensed for generalised anxiety disorder when symptoms have failed to be controlled by other medication. Dr Jagus informed us that he prescribed Pregablin due to the distress and anxiety exhibited by Mrs Allen. This medication was continued throughout her admission to Grianagh Court. There was a reduction in dosage in June, but following an escalation of her aggression, the medication was increased again to its previous dose with some resolution of symptoms. It is our opinion that the use of Pregablin could be justified.

(Not in the report, but significant. On 02 April 2012 and days earlier, Judith was presenting with suicidal ideation, yet Pregabalin's patient information leaflet details suicidal ideation as a side-effect, but the drug was still continued until 31 July 2012. It's known side-effects are irritability, memory impairment, depression, agitation, mood swings, difficulty finding words, hallucinations, aggression and mental impairment. It had been prescribed to Judith for at least eight months).

VII) Sodium Valproate. The licensed indications for this medication are all forms of epilepsy, migraine prophylaxis and mania. There is however, an evidence base for its use, with close monitoring of side-effects and response to severe behaviours that challenge in the context of dementia. Discussion with Dr Jagus was that this medication was prescribed due to Mrs Allen's increasing aggression and the risk she presented to others. It is our opinion that the use of Sodium Valproate could be justified in the clinical circumstances presented by Mrs Allen. However, it is our opinion that the use of Sodium Valproate should have been accompanied by a clear justification in the case notes as to why the medication was being used for an off-license indication, and in particular, what symptoms it was hoped that the medication would target, so that the decision could be made as to whether the medication was being of benefit.

(Not in the report, but significant: Sodium Valproate can precipitate Neuroleptic Malignant Syndrome, especially when used with antipsychotic drugs concurrently. (Ref. Clinical Psychopharmacology and Neuroscience 2017 Feb; 15.1.76. Author Veli Yildirim et al)

VIII) Risperidone. This medication is licensed as an antipsychotic and is the only atypical antipsychotic also licensed for the management of behavioural disturbances in dementia. Mrs Allen presented with intermittent auditory and visual hallucinations. The use of Risperidone for the treatment of these hallucinations was in our opinion appropriate. She also presented significant and challenging behavioural disturbance which was distressing for Mrs Allen and others. Low dose of Risperidone as prescribed for Mrs Allen was in our opinion an appropriate management of the behaviours. Close monitoring of response and side effects should have occurred. It is unclear from review of the notes what formal monitoring in these areas was occurring and difficult to determine whether the medication use beyond short-term use was purely for the treatment of visual and auditory hallucinations, or also for the management of behavioural disturbances.

The use of antipsychotic medication in patients with dementia does carry risks related to cerebrovascular adverse incidents. It is recognised good practice in view of these increased risks to clearly identify the potential harms and benefits of such medication in order that discussions can occur with the patient and their nearest relatives. All decisions need to be based on the best interests of the patient. It is our opinion that Mrs Allen's relatives should have been made fully aware of the risks and benefits of the medication and this should have been documented. It is our opinion that the failure to do so fell below standard of good practice. (Not in the report, but significant, was the lack of addressing the concomitant prescribing of risperidone and furosemide .... a diuretic..., and the ONLY diuretic known to further increase mortality in elderly dementia patients when co-prescribed with risperidone).

Diagnosis and Treatment of Delirium.

4.7 A formal diagnosis of delirium is not documented within the RiO healthcare records during Mrs Allen's admission to Grianagh Court. It is clear from the RiO records that during her last few days in Grianagh Court her presentation changed. She became physically less responsive and less able to care for herself. There was evidence of increase in temperature and a presumption of a urinary tract infection. On 16 of July 2012, Mrs Allen was noted to have recurrence of visual hallucinations and aggression. Risperidone was recommenced at this point. This would have been an appropriate treatment for visual hallucinations which had been a feature of her illness previously. It is not clear from the RiO records whether consideration was given at this point to delirium being the cause for her visual hallucinations.

4.8 On 20 July 2012, Mrs Allen's deteriorating physical condition prompted further investigation and a presumed diagnosis of urinary tract infection and pyelonephritis was made. Risperidone appears to have been continued at this point, although the reason for this is unclear from the records.

4.9 On 21 July in view of Mrs Allen's physical deterioration a medication review occurred. Plans were put in place to decrease and stop Pregablin and to omit Diazepam prescription. This was an appropriate adjustment in medication in view of the physical status of Mrs Allen. This rationalisation of medication was in our opinion an appropriate intervention for presumed delirium.

(Not in report, but significant: Judith was taking Pregablin and Diazepam still, when discharged back to Grianagh Court one week later. Clearly the plan was not implemented. No diagnosis of delirium was ever mentioned or noted in any records. Refer to report dated 11 December 2012, "Dr Jagus reviewed your mother's medication on 31 July 2012 and noted the diagnosis of cholecystitis. Due to your mother's drowsiness Dr Jagus discontinued the prescription of Pregablin and Risperidone and her Diazepam was reduced from 5mgs to 2mgs three times a day").

4.10 In summary, it is our opinion that Mrs Allen presented with a complex set of challenging and distressing symptoms which proved very difficult to control with the treatment interventions and medications available. The psychotropic medications prescribed fell within the range of medications appropriate for the diagnosis and symptoms presented by Mrs Allen. The combinations and dosages used were within acceptable parameters for the symptom combination described.

(Not in the report, but significant: if delirium, which is also a presentation in Neuroleptic Malignant Syndrome, was diagnosed, why were all the delirium inducing medications not stopped?).

4.11 It is our opinion that the lack of formal monitoring or recording of target symptoms when medications were introduced or doses were changed, resulted in difficulty assessing response and achieving appropriate dose titration. It is difficult from evidence available to be clear that non-pharmacological interventions were considered or used with Mrs Allen to determine their effectiveness.

Recommendations.

1. The hospital management and clinical leaders on Grianagh Court should set out guidance for staff in best practice for care planning. A system of clinical supervision and audit should be established to ensure that these standards are met.
2. Medical staff should ensure that their rationale and use of medication is appropriately documented, standards for monitoring set and appropriate discussion with patients and where appropriate relatives takes place to ensure consent.

5. Transfer of information Between Grianagh Court and the Medical Ward.

5.1 No letter documenting the transfer of care between Grianagh Court and the medical ward at Noble's could be found.

5.2 We discussed with Dr Jagus, Dr Balakrishnan and Dr Byrne the processes in place to ensure the safe handover of patients between the two hospitals. We were informed that the psychiatric and medical wards use different record systems. The mental health unit use an electronic patient record, the RiO system, to which the staff in medical wards have no access. We were informed that the arrangements for transferring information relies on telephone messages between members of staff, often junior doctors and nurses in the two hospitals.

6. Opinion: Diagnosis

6.1 It is our opinion that Mrs Allen had a diagnosis of dementia of the Alzheimer's type. This was a progressive disorder and, at the time of her death, the level of severity was severe.

6.2 Our reasons for concluding that the diagnosis was of dementia of the Alzheimer-type can be summarised as follows-

I) Mrs Allen's first presentation was with difficulties with memory and thinking. These were measurable on mental status testing which demonstrated progressive decline over time.

(Not in the report, but of significance; Judith first presented at Dr Jagus Out-Patient clinic with anxiety and depression, quote, "Indeed when she was first referred, it was difficult to assess her cognitive function because of the presence of significant depressive symptoms which were being treated at the time with Mirtazapine").

II) Mrs Allen required increasing care with regard to activities of daily living, including prompting for washing, dressing and eating. With time she needed significant assistance with all of these activities.

III) Mrs Allen demonstrated impaired visuospatial ability having difficulty recognising family and showed changes in personality and behaviour.

(Not in report, but significant: Judith never had any difficulty recognising family members).

IV) Mrs Allen's dementia was associated at times with auditory and visual hallucinations. These are known to be associated with Alzheimer's disease. (Not in report. These are commonly associated with Lewy Body Dementia).

6.3 There are no definitive diagnostic tests for Alzheimer's Disease. Mrs Allen had a CT scan and MRI scan documented in the notes but no reports were found. The CT scan is recorded in notes as being reported as normal. We assume that no changes were found on CT or MRI which would support a diagnosis other than Alzheimer's Disease without significant changes on a brain scan, as the pathology occurs at a cellular level.

6.4 We considered whether the Dementia was of a different type, for example Lewy Body Disease or Vascular Dementia. Mrs Allen's presentation was not typical of a vascular dementia. The progress of Vascular Dementia is typically a fluctuation stepwise progression of deficits, whereas Mrs Allen had a more progressive Dementia.

6.5 Although Mrs Allen had visual hallucinations which are a key feature of Lewy Body Dementia, she did not exhibit the other features of this type of dementia which include spontaneous Parkinsonian motor signs and fluctuation attention and concentration.

(Not in report, but significant: Judith presented early on in her dementia, significant sleep disturbances, where she was wandering at nighttime and going into other people's house. This insomnia/ sleep disturbances can be a key feature in Lewy Body Dementia. (Ref. www.lbda.org/10-things-you-should-know-about-lbd). (Dr Jagus prescribed Chloral Betaine 707mg to Judith for at least eight months for this problem).

6.6 Mrs Allen also had a diagnosis of delirium mixed picture (characterised by both hyper and hypoactive features). This started during the days preceding her transfer from Grianagh Court to Noble's Hospital on 25 July 2012 (error in report, was 20 July 2012). Our reasons for concluding this can be summarised as follows:-

1) Mrs Allen was at significant risk of developing delirium because of her age, the pre-existing diagnosis of dementia and the superimposed urinary tract infection, and presumed pyelonephritis. (Not in report, but highly significant – notably polypharmacy which carries a high risk of inducing delirium is not noted – Ref Postgraduate Medical Journal: An approach to drug induced delirium in the Elderly. Author K Alagiakrishnan 2004).

II) Mrs Allen's physical and mental state deteriorated with variable levels of consciousness and recurrence of visual hallucinations.

(Not in report, but significant: Judith had ongoing

problems with hallucinations and talking to children and animals since early 2011).

III) Mrs Allen presented as varying between agitated and restless and sedated and lethargic.

(Not in report, but significant: Both Dr Majheed and Dr Balakrishnan from the Medical Ward, described Judith as being in a coma-like state, both verbally and documented).

IV) It is possible that the symptoms of delirium persisted throughout her admission to Noble's Hospital and contributed to her difficulty eating and drinking and her requirements for increased physical care.

(Not in report, but significant: Judith had no difficulties eating, she point-blank refused to accept food. Her physical needs for care did not increase in Noble's Hospital, they began and stayed exactly the same as when she transferred from Grianagh Court on her first admission to the medical ward on 20 July 2012).

Delirium symptoms can continue for several months after causative factors such as infection have been fully treated. (Not in report, but significant: Delirium does not cover Judith's total inability to move; her lack of balance, to an extreme that she could not sit in a chair; her rigidity – noted when attempting lumbar puncture; Babinski signs, or her neck swelling and inability to swallow on her first transfer to Noble's Hospital, along with her lack of breathing compliance when being examined on that day).

7. Opinion: Did Mrs Allen have Neuroleptic Malignant Syndrome?

7.1 Neuroleptic Malignant Syndrome is a rare but serious side-effect of antipsychotic drugs. The symptoms are:-

I) Fever great than 38 degrees Celsius.

II) Muscle rigidity.

III) Autonomic instability, that is significantly fluctuating blood pressure and pulse rate.
IV) Altered consciousness.
(Not in report but significant: this is not an exhaustive list of symptoms relating to NMS, as detailed earlier, but Judith's temperature was 38.5 on 20 July, her admission day).

7.2 There is no diagnostic test for Neuroleptic Malignant Syndrome, but a raised creatine kinase is suggestive in combination with the clinical findings as outline in 7.1 above.

7.3 It is our opinion, very unlikely that Mrs Allen suffered from Neuroleptic Malignant Syndrome. We based this opinion on the following:-

1) Mrs Allen had been prescribed the neuroleptic drug, Risperidone for a period during April, May and part of June and did not develop any relevant symptoms. Although Mrs Allen was re-prescribed Risperidone on 16 July 2012 and developed a fever four days later, this fever was explained by the fact she had a significant kidney infection. There is no clinical reason to suppose that Mrs Allen had Neuroleptic Malignant Syndrome causing the fever.
(Not in the report but significant:- Risperidone was recommenced at 0.5mgs twice a day, then two days later it was increased to 1mg twice a day, even when a urinary infection was already identified which in itself can cause agitation and aggression in elderly people. This 0.5mg increase in Risperidone had not proven previously to be tolerated by Judith. It was reduced back down to 0.5mgs after two days. Later that evening Judith's severe incapacitation symptoms were noted. Judith was noted to have a tremor start on this day too. Pyelonephritis was ruled out by Consultant Physician Dr Joshi – he identified lower

UTI, but due to no urinalysis being undertaken, even the UTI was not proven).

II) There is no evidence that Mrs Allen had autonomic instability with fluctuations of blood pressure. She had an increased pulse rate due to infection. (Not in report, but significant. This was a presumed infection).

III) Although Mrs Quine described to us that her mother was stiff and rigid in the hours prior to her transfer to Noble's Hospital, this stiffness was not identified by medical staff in either Grianagh Court or the ward at Noble's. It is our opinion, on the balance of probabilities, that if rigidity had been a significant component of her clinical picture at the time, it would have been documented.

(Not in report but significant: Nurse Halsall at Grianagh Court noted swelling of the neck on 20 July 2012, with difficulty swallowing. Dr Nordgard noted her lack of chest compliance. Both would be typical of Neuroleptic Malignant Syndrome due to chest wall rigidity. (Ref Post Grad Journal 1998 1: 74:72-7 Author M Balza. Ref hospital physician.com Author TN Bottoni – 2002). Rigidity and inflexibility in Judith's legs was noted by Noble's staff when performing the lumbar puncture).

IV) It is our opinion, possible that Mrs Allen had developed stiffness or rigidity linked to the re-prescription of Risperidone. Although this was at a dose that had not caused stiffness in the past, her more fragile physical state may have caused stiffness which is a much more common side-effect of the Risperidone than Neuroleptic Malignant Syndrome. (Not in the report, but significant: I reported in my complaints letters that on 30 May 2012, when addressing my mother's bathroom needs, that I had noted her calf muscle looking extreme, and likened them to "footballers' legs". She was taking Risperidone concomitantly with Furosemide. Further research, due to my concern, discovered an article about a nurse who had been admitted to hospital, and medics later discovered that she had been taking 250mgs of Furosemide per day, to increase her muscle tone in her body. (Ref: Ruisz W et al, BMC Women's Health 2013). I also learned that Body Builders take Furosemide to release excess water from their body, to project muscle tone, especially in competitions. The fact that I noticed this in my mother, at a time when I had no access to her medical notes or prescribed medications was disturbing. The fact that my mother was only taking 20mg per day and this increased muscle tone was noticeable, would indicate to me, as a lay person, that some form of dehydration and/or metabolic phenomenon was occurring at that point in time).

VII) Mrs Allen did not have her creatine kinase checked which we believe the doctors would have done had they considered a diagnosis of Neuroleptic Malignant Syndrome even remotely likely.

(Not in report, but significant: Had the doctors in the medical ward received transfer notes explaining Judith's full history in the past week and detailing her total incapacitation, they may have been in a position to consider NMS. Delirium, a major component of NMS was never relayed from Mental Health Services to Medics).

7.4 It is our opinion, highly unlikely that Mrs Allen had an untreated Neuroleptic Malignant Syndrome which resolved on its own accord. This would have been highly unusual and atypical presentation which would in any event, have had no impact on Mrs Allen's subsequent prognosis as a resolved Neuroleptic Malignant Syndrome **does not have any long-term sequelae.**

(Not in the report, but highly significant: Neuroleptic Malignant Syndrome has been recorded many times by professionals as having residual catatonia, including negativism and refusal to eat, amongst other residual sequelae, following NMS. Some residual effects have been reported lasting up to six months after cessation of causative drugs. (Ref British Journal of Clinical Pharmacy Vol. 1 July/August 2009 Author E.Maule). Reports have been case noted where residual immobility and refusal to eat following a case of NMS, was successfully treated with twelve sessions of electroconvulsive therapy, following NMS. The patient regained mobility and commenced eating food again. (Ref Encephala 2005 Nov-Dec 2005;31(6 pt1) Author G. Benjellou et al). I can only conclude that if NMS had been considered and if Judith had been treated with ECT, when I raised the question on 07 September 2012 in the meeting, her outcome may have been different and her suffering less).

8. Opinion: Were the Staff at Noble's Hospital Given Sufficient Information for Mrs Allen's various conditions including delirium, when she was admitted in July 2012 to enable her to be treated appropriately?

8.1 It is our opinion that the responsibility for ensuring appropriate handover of care is a joint one between the discharging and receiving teams. The fact that the two relevant wards are on the same hospital site within a few hundred yards of each other, means there can be no reason why all the necessary information should not be made available to the new team looking after the patient.

8.2 It is our opinion that the current arrangement relies too much on possibly inexperienced junior doctors to provide all the relevant information that is necessary. There is no guidance in place as to the information that is needed. We believe that as the information is not provided in a written form to ensure that it is clearly understood what treatment the patient is on, why they are on it and the progress that they have made thus, **presents a significant risk to patient safety**.

8.3 It is our opinion there is no evidence that the failure of handover information in Mrs Allen's case resulted in poor or unsafe care.

We do believe, however, that the system in place does not offer sufficient safeguards for patient safety. (Not in the report, but significant: Really? Not poor or unsafe in Judith's case?).

Recommendations.

3. The medical admissions ward at Noble's Hospital should be able to access the RiO medical records for patients under their care.
4. A protocol should be drawn up of the standard expected for information transfer between the acute hospital and the mental health service. This process should be understood by all relevant staff involved and, in particular, junior doctors, doctors in training and locum doctors who will often be the clinicians responsible for implementing the guidelines.

9. Opinion: Capacity and Consent

9.1 We understand that capacity legislation has not yet been introduced in the Isle of Man. It is the case, however, that clinicians have a responsibility to ensure that where patients lack capacity, decisions are made in their best interests. The GMC sets out clear guidance about capacity as follows:-

"You must assess a patient's capacity to make a particular decision at the time it needs to be made. You must not assume that because a patient lacks capacity to make a particular decision on a particular case, they lack capacity to make any decisions at all.

If your decision leaves you in doubt about the patient's capacity to make a decision, you should seek advice from nursing staff or others close to the patient who may be aware of the patient's usual ability to make decisions and the particular communication needs".

9.2 In view of Mrs Allen's clear lack of capacity to consent to any management decisions, including prescription of medication, it should be expected that close relatives are engaged in decision making. It is impossible from the records to tell whether this occurred with any members of the multidisciplinary team. (not in the report, but significant is the fact that we stated no information as to Judith's medication was ever discussed during her admissions to Grainagh Court).

9.3 It is our opinion, and this was shared by Dr Jagus, that Mrs Allen lacked capacity to make decisions about medication when she was a patient in Grianagh Court. It is our opinion that because of Mrs Allen's lack of capacity, a discussion about medication and interventions used should have occurred within the multidisciplinary team, and with Mrs Allen's family. Dr Jagus informed us that this was his practice. It is unfortunate that there is no evidence of such discussions occurring in the case notes. It is our opinion that had this process been followed, it is likely that Mrs Allen's daughter would have been better able to understand both the severity of her mother's illness and the reasons why the medication used was being prescribed.

(Not in report, but significant: We as a family would have been at least aware of the increased mortality associated with Risperidone and the serious adverse side-effects and possible Neuroleptic Malignant Syndrome, along with the symptoms. We would have understood the two-fold further increase associated with the concomitant prescribing of Furosemide, and the serious risk of dehydration that could be involved).

5. The mental health team should institute guidance for best practice in assessing capacity and action required when capacity is lacking. This is necessary whether or not specific legislation is likely to be imminent; it would be sensible to wait to ensure such guidance is within the legal framework being introduced on the island.

10. This reiterates and details the 5 recommendations already detailed.

The report is signed by Dr Laurence Mynors-Wallis and Dr Cope.

My conclusions on receiving and reading the report were that Dr Jagus and the Mental Health team were falling far below standards expected and were not fit to recklessly prescribe such a shocking plethora of medications, evidenced by their admittance to not monitoring target symptoms of these medications; not providing transfer notes or communication with medical wards, and not informing our family of significant mortality risks and serious side-effects relating to such. Most importantly, was the failure to communicate to the medical ward, Dr Jagus' and the mental health unit's diagnosis of Judith's delirium, neck swelling, difficulty swallowing and tremor. All of which I could see only as a serious breach of duty and a serious risk to patient safety.

29
More Clarity

Further to receiving, and upon further perusal of this IRB report, I was very concerned by the bias and dismissal of the condition of Neuroleptic Malignant Syndrome, as if it were so rare, that it barely even existed.

I further researched the condition and found an article by author Dr Ryan Hall, a member of the Department of Psychiatry and Behavioural Sciences, John Hopkins, Baltimore, U.S. and who is a Clinical Professor of Psychiatry; Clinical Geriatrics, Vol. 14:5. May 2006.Neuroleptic Malignant Syndrome in the Elderly.

Excerpts from this are:-

"Neuroleptic and other dopamine-affecting agents are commonly used to treat a wide variety of psychiatric and non-psychiatric conditions in the elderly. With their increasing use, the rare but potentially lethal complication of Neuroleptic Malignant Syndrome (NMS) must be considered particularly in geriatric patients who are often taking multiple medications.

While this condition had been seen in patients of all ages, the elderly are particularly susceptible due to greater risk of dehydration, aging-related cognitive changes that may affect their dosing compliance, decreased dopamine activity that occurs naturally with aging. NMS is too often omitted from the differential diagnosis when elderly patients present with high fever, confusion and muscle stiffness.

Inciting of predisposing factors include dehydration, malnutrition, exhaustion, intramuscular injection of neuroleptics, advanced age, neuroleptic dose increases, dementia, anti-cholinergic agents and some antidepressants. It has been noted that the incidence of NMS increases during summer months, when the risk of dehydration is greatest.

It can occur following a single dose of any neuroleptic, or atypical neuroleptic. Neuroleptic Malignant Syndrome most characteristically develops 24-72 hours after the administration of a neuroleptic agent, or a change in dosage (usually an increase). Two-thirds of cases occur in the first week that a drug is administered. The duration of symptoms can last from 1 to 4 days, with most cases persisting for 1 to 14 days. Initially, there were few long-lasting reported sequelae of NMS following acute recovery. Case reports have recently documented neurological sequelae lasting months to years following resolution of initial NMS symptoms.

A complication of NMS can be anoxic brain damage".

After fully reading the findings of the IRB report and sending an e-mail to Andrea Roberts, IRB Clerk, I informed her that I was not fully satisfied, and questions still remained unanswered, along with some issues being factually inaccurate.

The Independent Review Body sent me a letter in reply, dated 27 January 2015:-

"Dear Mrs Quine
I am writing on behalf of the Panel in response to your e-mails and Mrs Andrea Roberts regarding the IRB, concerning the care of your late mother Mrs Judith Allen.

The IRB Panel members note that you cannot accept some of the findings of Dr Cope and Dr Mynors-Wallis and remain dissatisfied about some aspects of Mrs Allen's care/diagnosis.

I would however like to remind you that Andrew Guy (Panel Chairman) and I met you before the start of the hearing and explained the IRB Panels process and checked with you that you understood it, including the fact that the hearing and report concluded the process. It was our understanding that you accepted all of this.

The Panel fully considered your complaint at the Review Hearing, utilising the expertise of two highly qualified and experienced independent clinicians, and reached its conclusion as set out in the report. The experts are representatives of their respective Royal Colleges and the IRB are convinced that it is not possible to obtain a better standard of medical opinion anywhere in the British Isles.

Whilst we understand that you may feel that matters are still not fully resolved to your satisfaction, we must remind you that the IRB is obliged to work within the statutory framework set out by Tynwald (i.e. Isle of Man Parliament). This framework dictates that either the decision by a convenor (plus an appeal to a second convenor), OR a panel hearing is the end of the process. Therefore, the complaints procedure has now reached its end and there is no further recourse to resolution within the NHS framework.

Given all the above, we must respectfully advise you that we are not in a position to enter into any further correspondence on this matter, although we will ensure that you are informed of the outcome of the action plan at an appropriate time. We trust you will understand and accept this.

Yours sincerely
Vivienne Hare (IRB Convenor)".

Despite a few more attempts at conveying my points previously made, they refused to move on this stance. I wrote to politicians on the island, pointing out that not only was there inconclusive closure on my mother's death, but we, as a family, felt that our right to an inquest into Judith's death had been denied to us too.

Patient history had not been passed from Mental Health to the

Medical Ward, and the delirium diagnosis (a major component of NMS) was not conveyed beyond the coven of the mental health unit. This, from every angle of perspective, I could only see as gross negligence. As the Consultant Physicians explained on more than one occasion, there was "no medical explanation for Judith's condition".

I thought long and hard about the situation and came to the conclusion that this series of events must have affected previous dementia patients, and the most concerning outcome I could arrive at, was that it could happen again. I did not want another person, or family to experience this catastrophe again, so with this in mind, I took the decision to engage a lawyer, to present the evidence in an attempt to obtain a retrospective inquest, I knew it would be a long-shot and highly unusual, but I figured it would be worth a try. At the very least, I would have a detailed explanation and insight into how the Coroner would view the findings.

I had already been so concerned by the series of events that had occurred at the hospital; so much so, that when I discovered in December 2012, by way of another doctor looking at my hospital records, (just two months after my mother had died), that scan results from 2009 had not been fully disclosed to me, despite very distressing ongoing and painful symptoms, I took the decision to go off-island to Liverpool Women's Hospital for private treatment to undergo investigations, then underwent a full hysterectomy privately, in Liverpool too. That was the extent of my concern over clinical safety and integrity that I felt about Noble's Hospital, following my mother's death.

Had I not taken this step, I believe my problem would have persisted and the correct diagnosis never reached. I had multiple fibroids; one large, which my scans results showed but was relayed and detailed as essentially normal. The underlying cause of my pain, bleeding and frequent bathroom visits was a condition called adenomyosis, where the lining of the womb grows into the muscular wall of the womb causing bleeding and pain. The doctor performing the operation had explained to me later that the operation was quite difficult, due to the bulkiness of the uterus and womb. A small cyst that had been identified on my ovary, in a private scan done elsewhere, was not mentioned. My mother had been an ovarian cancer survivor and I was certainly not taking any risks. The complete hysterectomy meant a stress free, pain free, bleeding free life. I never looked back after that, yet the correct disclosure results at the time, would have led to further investigations and a timely diagnosis of the underlying cause.

With regards to Judith's death, I tried to engage with several lawyers on the island to present the case to the Coroner, but none were interested. One firm explained that they undertook work for the Department of Health and that it would be inappropriate for them to deal with the case.

The advocates that I eventually engaged, informed me that it would be a highly unusual case, but still, I outlined the case to the advocate and brought my full case notes into their office for photocopying.

I met the advocate once for the engagement meeting, then the next time was to bring the case file into their office. Most correspondence was by email. At £270 per hour for their fees, I hoped that many meetings were not necessary. My third meeting was to look at the submission document to be presented to the Coroner. I was to meet the advocate at 5.30pm at the Advocates offices. I arrived; the day was Friday. All the doors were locked and the lights were all switched off. I could see a faint light coming from underneath a door inside. I stood outside patiently in the drizzle. The advocate came to let me in, maybe ten minutes later. We went into a small office, where he presented the submission document. I started to read it; I must have looked up at him a couple of times, clearly shocked. Then remembering the £270 per hour he was charging me, I asked him what this sub-standard document was. It made very few of the serious points that I intended to highlight and was, without doubt, a half-arsed attempt to placate me.

I kept calm in my approach with him but expressed my concise opinion that I expected much more from a professional advocate.

It was, in my opinion, a document drawn up by a kid aspiring to be a lawyer. It reeked of resounding contempt towards me. I could not interpret it in any other way.

I took the document and explained that I would send a copy of what I wanted to be submitted to the Coroner, using the framework from the poorly drafted attempt.

I was fuming when I got outside of the office. He clearly did not want to undertake the task at hand, but I was paying for their service and I would insist they submitted a concisely constructed document requesting a retrospective inquest into Judith's death. At this point I deduced that an inquest would not happen, but I at least wanted the Coroner's input and perspective on the issues surrounding her death.

The final submission document and supporting documentation was sent to the Coroner, dated 9 February 2016.

On 20 May 2016, the Coroner replied to the advocate:

> Dear Mr ————
> Re The late Mrs Judith Anne Allen {Died 25 October, 2012} {Mrs Allen}.
>
> 1) I am now in a position to give a substantive response to your letter of 9 February 2016 regarding the request made on behalf of Mrs Victoria Quine (Mrs Quine) for an inquest to be held into the death of her late mother, Mrs Allen. I have taken the somewhat unusual step in this letter numbering the paragraphs for future reference by any interested person, or reviewing body.
> 2) May I firstly apologise for the delay in responding to you which has been due to me awaiting provision of the full medical and mental health records pertaining to Mrs Allen which were only received on 03 May 2016. I have now had a chance to carefully peruse such notes and records which have aided

me in reaching an informed view on the matter in hand. In making my decision I have also been assisted by your carefully drafted and very helpful outline submission dated 09 February 2016 together with the Supporting Bundle.

3) As you have set out, as Coroner of inquests I am duty bound to hold an inquest where there is reason to believe that a deceased died directly or indirectly, inter alia, as a result of negligence, misconduct or malpractice on the parts of others; or, in circumstances as may require investigation. (1) Despite in the current case the absence of a body, the interpretation of the terms set out in section 2(1)(6) of the Coroners of Inquests Act 17 (the 17 Act) is key to my decision upon Mrs Quine's request. I am not aware of any Manx case-law regarding interpretation of section 2(1)(b) of the 17 Act. My interpretation of the relevant terms is as follows:

4) The term "negligence" in relation to a hospital death includes advice, act or omissions in the course of the clinicians professional work which no member of the profession who was reasonably well-informed and competent would have given or done or omitted to do, and includes an error "such as" no reasonably well-informed and competent member of that profession could have made (2). It appears that there is clear overlap in respect of "negligence" with terms "misconduct" and "malpractice". A mere act of negligence is not necessarily misconduct as such usually involves something more serious.(3).

5) As to the meaning of the term "reason to believe", I interpret that as meaning a knowledge of facts from which a reasonable man would arrive at the relevant belief. Facts from which a reasonable man might suspect the relevant conclusion cannot be enough. (4) In my view the test is that it must be shown from the facts that it is reasonably likely as opposed to being fanciful, that negligence, misconduct or malpractice caused or contributed to the death. Likewise, a mere possibility is insufficient (5).

6) As to the term "died directly or indirectly as a result of" imputes the requirement of causation. There must be reasonable grounds to believe that an act of negligence, misconduct or malpractice has caused or contributed to the death but it certainly does not need to be the sole cause of death.
7) I have reminded myself of the concept of the duty to hold an inquest into a death in such circumstances as may require investigation (7) and the link to the state's duty of inquiry where a death engages a deceased's right to life under Article 2 of the European Convention on the Human Rights. I have analysed the state's duties in previous cases (8). I have reminded myself of the power to hold an inquest where (inter alia) the Coroner has reason to believe that the death occurred in the Island, but the body cannot be recovered and there is reason to believe that the deceased died, inter alia, as a result of negligence, misconduct or malpractice (9). The discretion is to be exercised judicially. My starting point therefore must be the recorded cause of death.
8) For brevity, I do not need to set out a full chronology of events; a short chronology can be gleaned from reading, as I have, the relevant 50 pages of the Mental Health Services (MHS) computerised RIO system records from 2009, and the over 1300 pages of medical records including the Clinical and Nursing Notes from Nobles and Ramsey Cottage Hospital mostly from 2012. I accept that the broad factual circumstances are as follows:-

    I) Mrs Allen was aged 70 years old at the date of death.
    II) Mrs Allen started to encounter depressive symptoms and memory problems which were sufficient to be reported to MHS in the latter part of 2008 and then was diagnosed with **Probable** Alzheimer's-Type Dementia in 2010.
    III) By October 2011, family circumstances including Mrs

Allen's husband suffering a stroke meant that Mrs Allen could not be cared for at home. Mrs Allen's daughter was unable to cope with her mother due to Mrs Allen's aggressive outbursts and severe mood swings.

IV) Mrs Allen was initially placed at Grianagh Court on an emergency basis and then in December 2011 moved to Laxey Glen House Residential Home, but after only approximately two months moved to Beaconsfield Towers Nursing Home as the staff in the residential home in Laxey were struggling to cope. It was a similar situation at Beaconsfield and Mrs Quine confirms that her mother's behaviour could at times be extreme and disruptive.

V) On 2 April 2012, Mrs Allen was admitted "under Section" to Grianagh Court for assessment. She was discharged from "section" by the end of April 2012 but remained a voluntary inpatient at Grianagh Court. Whilst in Grianagh Court Mrs Allen suffered advancing behavioural and psychological symptoms of Dementia including significant hostility and aggression to others. Mrs Allen was prescribed anti-psychotic medication including Risperidone from 02 April 2012. The Risperidone was reduced on 11 June 2012 and ceased to be administered on 18 June 2012. The quantity of dosage was within BNF guidelines, but the duration of dosage for treatment was in excess of the 6 week guideline.

VI) Risperidone was re-started again on 14 July 2012 and increased on 16 July 2012 by the locum Psychiatrist Dr O'Sullivan as Mrs Allen had exhibited increased agitation and aggressive behaviour.

VII) On 19 July 2012 the staff at Grianagh Court noted that Mrs Allen appeared slightly drowsy and unsteady on her feet. Mrs Allen's mobility continued to decline and she was noted to have a tremor when trying to drink. The Risperidone dose was reduced to the previous level.

VIII) On 20 July 2012 it was noted that Mrs Allen was very drowsy. She did drink a glass of juice. Her medication was withheld. She had rashes on both shins. She was medically examined on the afternoon of 20 July 2012 and found to have a temperature of 37.5 degrees Celsius, (Not in report, but Judith's MH notes detail 38.5 degrees Celsius later that same day). She was reported as not responding adequately. On examination by Dr Nordgard there was a dry tongue and mucous membranes. The medical impression was a potential fever of unknown origin and dehydration.

IX) The family noted that there was swelling around Mrs Allen's face and neck and on admission to Noble's on 20 July and she had a high temperature. On admission her urea and creatine electrolytes levels were normal indication that there was no clinical dehydration. A kidney infection was diagnosed (pyelonephritis) and Mrs Allen was prescribed I/V antibiotics.

X) Mrs Allen was transferred back to Grianagh Court on 27 July 2012. But was unable to tolerate fluids.

XI) Mrs Allen was transferred to the medical ward at Noble's on 28th July 2012 and subsequently a diagnosis of cholecystitis was made.

XII) Mrs Allen's Risperidone prescription was terminated on 31 July 2012.

XIII) Mrs Allen remained an inpatient in Noble's until mid-October 2012, her gall bladder infection was treated with IV antibiotics, however her level of consciousness and willingness/ability to eat remained poor. Mrs Allen lost weight. Efforts at artificial nutrition were not successful and in mid-September dislodged the PEG tube that had been surgically inserted and a clinical decision in the patient's best interests was taken not to re-site the tube. Following consultation with the family in mid-September 2012, a decision was taken that Mrs Allen was to receive palliative care.

XIV) On 15 October 2012, Mrs Allen was transferred to Ramsey Cottage Hospital for palliative care and the Care Plan Index referred to Mrs Allen suffering from End-Stage dementia. Mrs Allen was placed on the Liverpool Care Pathway on 22 October 2012 following assessment by Dr Allinson.

XV) Mrs Allen died 25 October 2012. The medical cause of death was given as 1(a) Dementia and 1(b) Essential Hypertension.

9) The above chronology does not really give a full picture of the case. Over the last four days I have almost exclusively spent my time reviewing in careful details the medical records regarding Mrs Allen. It is a cheerless record indicating the unenviable advance of a progressive, pernicious and highly challenging natural disease in circumstances where, to my mind on the information before me, very little could have been done by either Mrs Allen's family or the medical profession to lessen the effects of mental degeneration in a person who was only just passed retirement age.

10) The records of MHS refer to the onset of cognitive difficulties in terms of Mrs Allen's memory from late 2008. In September 2010 the diagnosis referred to by the specialist Consultant Psychiatrist, Dr Jagus in his letter to Mrs Allen's GP, Dr Allinson was "Probable Alzheimer's-Type Dementia…ICD Code – F00-1". I shall set out below the fact that the Independent expert evidence before me corroborates the diagnosis.

11) The Deceased's husband, Mr Allen, clearly bore the burden of looking after his wife lovingly and stoically until October 2011, which was well past the normal point that the professionals should step in. From evidence there seems to be no doubt that by that stage Mrs Allen was suffering from a severe form of Dementia and such significantly worsened in the months thereafter.

12) As I understand the position Mrs Quine disputes the primary cause of death listed on the MCD being Dementia. Instead it is submitted that there are reasonable grounds to believe that Mrs Allen died as a result of Anorexia due to residual catatonia caused by Neuroleptic Malignant Syndrome (NMS), arising through the negligent prescription/monitoring of Risperidone and other psychotropic medication in the period April 2012 to July 2012.
13) I have carefully read the medical articles and papers that are included in the Bundle of Key Documents that you provided to me. However, I am not aware of there being any case-specific admissible expert evidence submitted in support of Mrs Quine's request for an inquest and/or refuting the cause of death provided by Dr Allinson in October 2012 in the form of the Medical Certificate of Cause of Death, which was submitted by Mrs Quine when acting as the informant during the registration of death process.
14) The only case-specific medical evidence before me is in the form of the expert report of the independent psychiatrists Dr Mynors-Wallis and the Dr Denise Cope dated 23 October 2014. It is clear that their expert opinion is that Mrs Allen was suffering from Dementia of the Alzheimer's-type which was at a severe form at the time of her death and such lends significant weight to the registered cause of death. I have noted your suggestion that the emphasis of a coroner's inquiring regarding a cause of death is different to the terms of reference of the Independent Review Body (IRB) which was charged with investigating Mrs Quine's complaint which required an investigation into the issue of Mrs Allen's medical care. Although I recognise the overall difference in focus, the specific areas of investigation particularly of the independent experts reporting to the IRB was very much covering the same ground that would concern me as a Coroner if an inquest was to be held

and therefore likewise is highly informative in respect of my deliberations at this stage.

15) As to lack of definitive diagnosis of Alzheimer's Disease, Mrs Quine points to the lack of any positive results in terms of any test for the disease and in her manuscripts comments upon the independent experts' report, has indicated that her mother received a letter in 2011 indicating that there were "no signs of Alzheimer's". The experts communicated that patients can suffer Alzheimer's Disease without significant changes on the brain scan. I accept that view.

16) Mrs Quine hypothesised that Mrs Allen may have been suffering from undiagnosed Lewy Body Dementia (LBD) instead of Alzheimer's Disease and I have read the articles supplied in the bundles in support of such a conclusion. However, such articles in my view are no substitute for expert evidence. The independent experts in this case have discounted the evidence of LBD. They opine that although the presence of visual hallucinations in Mrs Allen was indicative of the condition, LBD was unlikely because Mrs Allen did not exhibit the other features of that type of dementia, including spontaneous Parkinson motor signs and fluctuating attention and concentration. I have noted that the reference Mrs Quine makes to Mrs Allen having a shuffling gate (sic) and tremors on 19 July 2012, but in respect of the observation of tremor that was isolated to the acute phase of the illness which Mrs Allen was suffering in mid July 2012. There is no mention of significant symptoms of motor skill abnormality elsewhere in the RIO notes and Mrs Allen's mobility on the various CPA Assessments over the time that her cognitive abilities were deteriorating in 2010 onwards make no mention of motor signs or poor mobility. Indeed, the physical condition of Mrs Allen, in terms of being a strong mobile person unfortunately added to the risks that Mrs Allen posed to others at the time of her

compulsory admission to Grianagh Court under section 2 Mental Health Act at the beginning of April 2012.

17) As to the suggestion that Mrs Allen suffered NMS, I have noted Mrs Quine's hypothesis that such manifested over a significant period of time from Mrs Allen being first prescribed Risperidone in early April 2012. However, clear medical opinion is that NMS is an acute illness rather than one of chronic aetiology and manifestation. The independent experts formed the view that it was very unlikely that Mrs Allen suffered from NMS in July 2012. Mrs Quine has referred to the prescription of the antimuscarinic drug, Procyclidine by the F2 doctor on 19 July 2012 as indicating a possibility of a drug induced dystonic reaction. Furthermore, Mrs Quine points to Mrs Allen having swelling in her neck from 20 July 2012 and difficulty swallowing on 28 July 2012. Mrs Quine also points to the loss of mobility of Mrs Allen in terms of ability to walk, talk, eat and drink prior to hospitalisation on 20 July 2012 and the recording of Babinski sign in the clinical notes from 02 August 2012. Nonetheless, it is clear that the independent medical experts had access to the clinical information referred to in the notes. The experts gave an apparently logical rationale for their opinion ruling out NMS as being likely. In particular, I note that the experts based their decision on the following-

a) There had been no adverse reaction to Mrs Allen to Risperidone when previously prescribed from April 2012 to mid-June 2012. The development of fever in or around 20th July was explained by the independently verified significant kidney infection. The experts indicated that there was no clinical reason to suppose NMS caused fever. Furthermore, in this regard I have reviewed the medical records regarding the level of pyrexia and such indicates the temperature profile did not follow that expected in a diagnosis of NMS.

b) There was no evidence of autonomic instability of blood pressure or pulse rate. In this regard Mrs Quine refers to her poor breathing being noted, but such is not specifically highlighted in the vital signs record in terms of respiration rate or blood oxygen saturation levels.

c) The experts considered Mrs Quine's anecdotal evidence of stiffness and rigidity in the hours before admission to Noble's. Nonetheless, they noted that such symptoms had not been identified by clinical or nursing staff in either establishment at this time.

   It seems to me that the experts adopted a logical approach in concluding that if the characteristic lead-piping symptom had existed in Mrs Allen, it would have been identified by staff in either the mental health or medical setting. In any event the expert opinion was that, even if there was such stiffness linked to the re-prescription of Risperidone, it was much more likely a symptom of Mrs Allen's more fragile physical state through the common side-effect of Risperidone, rather than NMS.

d) The experts considered it highly unlikely that NMS would resolve of its own accord. They referred to it being rare but a significant medical emergency. They concluded that the presentation of Mrs Allen in the context of what is known of NMS would have been highly unusual and atypical.

18) I accept such conclusions. I do note that in respect of the experts' reference to there being no long-term sequelae of NMS, Mrs Quine suggests that this is wrong. I agree with her view in light of the NHS Medicines Q & A's on NMS on 03 February 2014, which refers to, "A significant minority of patients suffer long-term sequelae including neurological impairment, muscle contraction and cognitive defects". However, such error does not appear to me to undermine the expert's overall conclusion that NMS was not present in Mrs Allen. Mrs Quine alleges residual catatonia as being the long-term sequelae in her mother's case. However, there has been no expert evidence to indicate that such is a well observed recognised consequence of NMS.

19) I have noted the reference to a small increase in risk due to concomitant prescription of Furosemide and Risperidone and the anecdotal evidence of dehydration, but there is no empirical evidence of dehydration.
20) The experts opined that delirium was the far more likely explanation for the altered consciousness of Mrs Allen. I note that in reaching that conclusion the experts had borne in mind that delirium was not recorded at the time of admissions or thereafter as a "formal classification of symptoms". However, the experts conclude that Mrs Allen had a "diagnosis of delirium mixed picture" (Characterised by both hyper and hypoactive features)". Such conclusion was based on:
    a) Mrs Allen being at a significant risk of suffering delirium based on her age, her dementia and the urinary tract infection, presumed pyelonephritis.
    b) Mrs Allen's physical and mental state deteriorated with variable levels of consciousness and reoccurrence of visual hallucinations.
    c) Mrs Allen's state varied between agitation/restlessness and sedated/lethargic.
    d) it being probable that delirium persisted throughout Mrs Allen's admission to Nobles and such features would continue for several months after the causative factors have been fully treated.
21) I am a little confused at the references to catatonia being the cause of Mrs Allen not eating, when it is suggested by Mrs Quine that Mrs Allen chose not to eat. It seems to me far more likely that the lack of ability to eat was a result of dementia itself whether directly or through the residual effects of delirium. The attempts at self-withdrawal of the nasogastric feeding tube and, more seriously the PEG tub were in my view far more likely due to dementia rather than catatonia.
22) As stated in the absence of any case-specific expert opinion to the contrary, I am of the view that it has not been established

that there is any reason to believe that NMS was the cause of Mrs Allen's death. Indeed, it appears on the evidence before me that the cause of death was an entirely natural one, namely dementia.

23) I have noted criticisms Mrs Quine has raised regarding the clinical team's care of Mrs Allen and in particular the level of recorded/monitoring of the effects of medication upon her and a detailed care plan as to her treatment. I have noted the content of the complaint regarding the lack of consultation with the next of kin and the complaint regarding the following of the Liverpool Care Pathway as to the palliative care that was provided to Mrs Allen in her last days. It is clear that the Review Panel found a good deal of room for improvements in term of the recommendations made. However, the suggestions that such is highly indicative of negligence is a matter of considerable debate. In reading the records of Mrs Allen's treatment it is clear that most unfortunately she was suffering very severe Dementia of the most distressing sort. There is no cure for Dementia and the ability to control Mrs Allen's symptoms in the year before her death was a significant challenge to medical professionals. In such circumstances it is by no means clear in terms of there being reason to believe that the actions of two very experienced psychiatrists, namely Dr Jagus and Dr O'Sullivan in trying to treat the worsening aggression, disruptive and potentially dangerous behaviour of Mrs Allen's in Grianagh Court in the early summer of 2012, fell below the standard of the competent and informed professional. That said, even if a breach of duty of care could be established as set out above, the causative link of any alleged negligence to the death has not been established. It therefore follows that the existence of any perceived short-comings in care do not obligate the Coroner to hold an inquest.

24) I have considered your additional submissions on the basis that irrespective of the issue of the cause of death, Mrs Allen's

death was in circumstances which are such as to require investigation. In this respect you raise the provision of Article 2 of the ECHR and the state's duties thereunder. For reasons given above, I do certainly not find that there is reason to believe that Mrs Allen's death was as a result of negligence. For the same reason there is even less room for suggestion of a neglect verdict, as that term is known in its limited coronial context. Furthermore, the same difficulty regarding the causation arises, as set out above. Mrs Allen's medical condition was complex in respect of an incurable and very advanced form of dementia. In my view there is no real evidence as to there being a basic step in provision of medical care which if taken would have significantly prolonged Mrs Allen's life.

25) I am aware that a large amount of time has passed since the death. Mrs Quine did not alert the Coroner at the time of her mother's death regarding any of these issues which has meant no postmortem has been held whereby the condition of Mrs Allen's brain at cellular level is known. It appears to me that the inquest would merely go over the same ground covered by the IRB incurring further significant costs and from what I have seen thus far there seems to be very little prospect of advancing matters beyond the finding of the IRB.

26) For the reasons already advanced, I do not see that I am under a duty to hold an inquest. As to the discretion to hold an inquest, I consider that it would not ultimately be in the public interest to pursue that course in circumstances where the death occurred a significant time ago, where concluded that there is no reason to believe that the death was unnatural or that it involved a gross failure on the part of the state to provide basic medical care, which would have averted the death.

27) Of course, I understand the disappointment that my decision will cause to Mrs Quine. I have noted that she had obviously spent a vast amount of time researching the matter, but such

research is no substitute for proper expert evidence. I will of course keep an open mind such, that if highly qualified case-specific medical expert evidence in the form of an expert's report was provided to me indicating that NMS was a definite causative factor in Mrs Allen's death, I would look into the matter again, but as things stand, I must decline Mrs Quine's request to hold an inquest.

Thank you for your attention.
Yours sincerely
J.A. Needham
Coroner of Inquests"

30
The Finale

Sometimes, I wished that I did not have the need for so many questions to be answered, but I still did. Although I accepted the Coroner's decision to not hold a retrospective inquiry, I still felt compelled to write to the Coroner again, through the Advocate.

My letter was dated 31 May 2016. Excerpts are as follows:-

"Dear Coroner Needham

Re: Mrs Judith Anne Allen

Thank you for your letter dated 20 May 2016 with regards to a request for a retrospective inquest into my late-mother's death.

I respect your decision on this request, yet before closure is complete, I would like to raise a few outstanding issues, with regards to your comments and reasons stated for not undertaking the requested inquiry.

I have firstly referred to the issues correlating to your numbered paragraphs, for ease of use and for future reference.

With regards to paragraph 4, referring to the term "negligence" in relation to a hospital death. We, as a family, believe that not ensuring that full patient history and notes were given to the new ward from the mental health unit, (this would include the expert independent assessors'' psychiatric opinion that the patient was at high risk of delirium), was an act of negligence, placing the patient in imminent danger. Particular mention of the patient's total lack of capacity within twenty four hours, whilst at the mental health unit was necessary. Without the information and history, no detection of delirium was possible, and no urinalysis was performed to detect such delirium. Having a medical records system "RIO" in the mental health ward that was not accessible to the medical ward, again must be a failure, classed as detrimental to the patient's treatment and health. "Polypharmacy" had been noted previous by Dr Slater, as a danger to the patient. Polypharmacy – a well-known cause of delirium, especially in dementia patients. Therefore, it would not have been unreasonable to have expected the expert opinion of a Consultant Pharmacist, upon Judith's admission to hospital. Sadly, a role that was not in place at either the mental health unit, or at the hospital, at the time of the patient's admission and death.

Referring to your paragraph 7, where a death engages a deceased's right to life under

Article 2 of the ECHR, with reference to the above points made, we believe there was a breach of this Act under Article 2.

With regards to paragraph 12, surrounding the primary cause of death, detailed on the death certificate as "Dementia". I am disputing this for the above reasons also, and for the added fact that we were informed, verbally, at a meeting one which was recorded), by the very experienced Consultant psychiatrist, Dr Jagus, that the deceased was in the "early stages of dementia". The hospital was informed by the same Consultant psychiatrist, by written correspondence that Judith was in the "early stages of dementia" too. Why was this? Just weeks before her death. This is in direct conflict with the death certificate. The G.P. who signed this certificate was not a dementia specialist. Therefore, he must have taken advice and direction from the same Consultant Psychiatrist, Dr Jagus. Why have these concerns not been addressed?

With reference to paragraph 14, regarding "the only case-specific independent medical evidence before me is in the form of the expert report of the independent psychiatrists Dr Laurence Mynors-Wallis and Dr Denise Cope". I think it is important to highlight that when the pre-arrangements for convening the IRB were underway, I was advised that the Independent Assessors would be appointed through the Royal Colleges – plural. It would have been reasonable to have expected one of those to be the Royal College of Physicians.

Regarding paragraph 1, where you identify an error in the independent Assessors report, saying that, "However such error does not appear to me to undermine the experts overall conclusion that NMS was not present in Mrs Allen". I allege that this "error" demonstrates a deliberate act of providing a misleading statement, to support and defend their fellow psychiatrist. Two experts in the field of Old Age Psychiatry cannot innocently make such a mistake. This demonstrates a clear undermining of the integrity of their report". End

I never expected anymore from this process of requesting a retrospective inquest, but it did prove to me that there was a certain amount of white-washing that was happening.

What startled me further, was after collecting my original files from the Advocates offices, I noticed sometime after, that the hospital letter dated 29 January 2013, was completely missing. It was an overall huge file that I had left for photocopying, so there was a little room for error. Thankfully, all documents had been scanned and backed up too. Yet, the fact that the letter was missing, highlighted a few major factors within the report. These were:-

On 20 July 2012 (the day of first medical ward admission), "RN Halsall attempted to assist your mother in taking fluids, but she was unable to swallow".

"Later that same afternoon, RN Halsall noted that your mother's neck was swollen". (The swelling that I described many times, but which had no depression when the skin was pressed. The "unable to swallow", was probably due to this neck swelling. The very swelling that had been denied was present or documented, throughout the complaints process).

On 28 July 2012 at 16.17 hours, RN Dela Rosa (who worked with my mother most closely), asked the duty doctor to review your mother. RN Dela Rosa was concerned about your mother's overall condition. Dr Zaijka attended the ward and examined your mother. Your mother was then transferred to the Medical Assessment Unit (MAU) at Noble's hospital. It was at this point that HCA Moore noticed your mother's neck was swollen".

More concerning, this is the swelling documented in the hospital letter and noted by staff, yet not documented in the Mental Health notes and never passed onto the medical ward. I surmise that if Medics were unfamiliar with the patient, then they may not have been able to identify that swelling, due to the "non-depression of the skin" that I described. It was not normal swelling. This neck swelling; inability to swallow; temperature of 38.5 degree Celsius; mutism; total incapacitation; lack of chest compliance, sweating and racing pulse that were noted at Grianagh Court, needed passing from Mental Health to the Medical Ward. Diagnosis of UTI or Pyelonephritis was made on the basis of the assumption of a continuing urine infection and the presence of leukocytosis. Leukocytosis is a major component of Neuroleptic Malignant Syndrome, as is delirium, which again, was a diagnosis from Mental Health, which was never passed to the Medics.

Further to this, the letter states, "It would appear that you are correct and the Risperidone was not stopped on admission".

I later complained to the Advocates Office about what I believed to be mis-advice and poor service from them. They replied to me with an offer of reducing the bill by thousands, leaving me with a final bill of over ten thousand pounds. I readily accepted, as no other outcome would be beneficial. A legal deadline had been missed, and no amount of complaining would bring this back.

What will always stay with me through Judith's hospital stay is the fact that the Consultant Physician explained that there was "no medical reason for your mother's condition". She was in the medical ward for nearly three months, during which time, delirium was never mentioned by the medics as a cause of Judith's immobility and refusal to eat. Delirium that is a major symptom of NMS.

What was startlingly evident too, was the fact that the Consultant Psychiatrist, Dr Jagus, went from a diagnosis of "very early, well early stages dementia, be it rapidly progressing", to "advanced dementia" in less than one month. The delirium diagnosis has only ever been diagnosed by Dr Jagus too. What is most concerning, is the dementia diagnosis of "Probable Alzheimer's Type Dementia" and then without a further thought or an ounce of caution, subjected Judith to a reckless prescription of medications, without any monitoring or recording of symptoms or possible side-effects of the medication; never questioning if the prescribed drugs were actually making her worse; prescribing off-label and without any caution with regards to the high risk of mortality associated with them. Not informing, or discussing the medication, and associated risks demonstrated a high level of complacency and contempt towards Judith and our family.

The Lewy Body Dementia Association in the United States details Lewy Body Dementia as the second most common dementia after Alzheimer's Disease and is often misdiagnosed as such. They quote on their website:-

"While the symptoms of LBD maybe similar to Alzheimer's and Parkinson's Disease, the treatment strategy is more challenging, because fewer medications can be used safely, warns Howard I. Hurtig M.D., Chair, Department of Neurology, Pennsylvania Hospital and member of the LBDA Scientific Advisory Council.. "I cannot overemphasise the need to avoid medications that can worsen the symptoms of LBD. Every patient with this disease and their caregivers should be familiar with the list of acceptable and forbidden drugs". End.

I would truly like to see the use of Risperidone stopped in elderly, dementia patients. In my experience the risks are just not worth taking, especially with the evidence that the standards and good practice guidelines recommended are being ignored.

One of the most recent insights into Lewy Body Dementia, is a really emotive and sad series of videos, depicting Joe with his mother

Molly who has LBD on Youtube, called "Mollysmovement.com". The facial expressions and frustrations that I see are so typical of how Judith was in 2011. I am, since seeing these videos, convinced that it was Lewy Body Dementia that Judith suffered from, especially combined with the night-time episodes with Judith that were draining my father of his sleep. In their nearly fifty years of marriage, it was the first time that they had slept in separate bedrooms. Sometimes my father said that Judith scared him, when she came into his bedroom at night and had strange conversation with him, or she would be shouting at him for not apparent reason.

Polypharmacy must be impossible to monitor in these people, who cannot converse concisely. It is at worst, "chemical torture". One drug, one reaction must be the way forward. This vulnerable section of society need protecting against such abusive prescribing practices. Risperidone should be banned totally for dementia patients. The side-effects are far too hideous.

The pharmaceutical industry has a lot to answer for too, and it has not gone unnoticed. In the US criminal proceedings were taken by the Government against, the pharmaceutical company Janssen, a subsidiary of Johnson & Johnson, who were promoting the antipsychotic Risperdal (risperidone), medicines to elderly dementia patients by urging the prescribers' to use Risperdal to treat symptoms such as anxiety, agitation, depression, hostility and confusion, which was an unapproved use, rendering the product misbranded. Back-handers and commissions were being paid to promote risperidone to these patients. Janssen pleaded guilty and will pay a total in $400 million, which includes the criminal fine of $334 million. (ref www.justice.gov/opa/pr/johnson-johnson-pay-more-22-billion-resolve-criminal-and-civil-investigations).

Johnson & Johnson are under further criminal investigation for concealing the cancer risk of their baby powder that allegedly contains asbestos and which causes a form of ovarian cancer. J & J has been sued more the thirteen thousand times already. Who can be trusted?

Just from my experience, Psychiatry needs to address their failings and prove themselves to be a profession of integrity, rather than making mere assumptions, followed by a "suck it and see" approach to care planning.

The UK Government, under The National Dementia Strategy for England, commissioned Professor Sube Banerjee to compile a report on the use of antipsychotic medication in dementia patients.

"A Report for the Minster of State for Care Services by Professor Sube Banerjee – **Time for Action**".

Extracts from his letter dated 03 October 2009, to the Minster states:-

"I was asked last year to examine the use of antipsychotic medication for people with dementia in the NHS in England and this is my review:-"

"There have been increasing concerns over the past years about the use of these drugs in dementia. The findings of my review confirm that there are indeed significant issues in terms of quality of care and patient safety. These drugs appear to be used too often in dementia and, at their likely level of use, potential benefits are most probably outweighed by their risk overall".

"We need to make reductions in the use of these medications a clinical governance priority across the NHS, with strong national, regional and local leadership from the Department of Health, the Care Quality Commission, strategy health authorities, primary care trusts (PCTs), mental health trusts and acute trusts. We need a cycle of audit that will deliver good quality information on the use of these drugs in dementia safely and drive up the quality of initiation, monitoring and maintenance of these medications when they are needed".

In Part 2 – **Findings**:-

This includes comments from professionals and carers about antipsychotic medication. One such comments reads:-

"I hold them responsible for his rapid loss of speech, the constant drooling, his mask-like frozen expression, the constant jerking of his right foot that stayed with him for the rest of his life, and rapid onset of incontinence. While still able to walk, he would walk leaning over sideways or backwards at an alarming angle, and no doubt it was this, 'unbalancing', that caused the hip fractures. Soon he developed epileptic fits and I cannot be sure that it was not related to the antipsychotic".

Another reads:-

"At 5pm precisely I have to give her medication: warfarin and (an antipsychotic). Within half an hour the change in her is drastic. On one occasion she was slumped sideways and fainted. She cannot move or talk properly and we virtually have to carry her into the car to take her back. They had been described previously as, 'to take the edge off the Alzheimer's. To be frank I am now worried to death at the consequence of them".

The report also details, "Typical antipsychotic are associated with common and serious adverse effects, including over-sedation, hypotension, involuntary movements, (including irreversible late onset tardive dyskinesia), Parkinsonian symptoms (rigidity, tremor and problems with walking and the rare occurrence of the cardio toxicity (damage to the heart), high fever and vascular collapse (neuroleptic malignant syndrome). Since their introduction, the use of the atypical antipsychotic has become much more common than the typicals, due to their generally favourable side-effect profile, with the incidence of Parkinsonian side-effects and tardive dyskinesia much lower for atypical antipsychotics.

In Section 2.3 **Concerns Regarding the Safety of Antipsychotic Drugs in People with Dementia.**

He cites, "People with dementia may well fall into a high-risk group for side-effects on the basis of age, frailty, physical co-morbidity and interactions with other drugs being taken. It has become clear that people with dementia, as a whole are at a higher risk of potentially serious adverse effects from antipsychotic medication".

The full Banerjee report can be found at www.jcpmh.info/wp-content/uploads/time-for-action.pdf

Neuroleptic Malignant Syndrome is a rare, but potentially lethal complication of neuroleptics – most literature states that. Yet, if incidents of NMS in dementia patients go undiagnosed, untreated and unreported, I have a strong suspicion that it is probably more common in elderly dementia patients on polypharmacy and other complications, than it is rare, due to being recorded merely as "advanced dementia" and blinkering the real truth/diagnosis.

In Judith's case the Psychiatrist changing his diagnosis from, "early stages of dementia, be it rapidly progressing", to "advanced and last stage dementia", in a time period of just over one month is not acceptable. The question is, how often does this happen to other dementia patients? We had considered in Judith's case, that the preliminary diagnosis maybe wrong and we asked for a "second opinion". The fax request was written out, but never faxed across. We can only therefore conclude that it is a blatant case of changing the diagnosis to fit the symptoms. Not informing the next of kin to Judith, about her medication regime and the increased risks of mortality and side-effects of the medication, when she lacked the capacity for consent, must render the Psychiatrist individually, and the Isle of Man Hospital and Government jointly responsible for Judith's safety. The fact that her Consultant Psychiatrist wrote a letter telling the Hospital Management that he could find no interaction information between Risperidone and Furosemide is tremendously concerning, when the Patient Information Leaflet clearly states that concomitant use of Risperidone with Furosemide increases mortality in elderly dementia patients, nearly doubling the risk, when compared to Risperidone solely – let alone allowing for a wrong diagnosis of the dementia type too. Is this a doctor who should be in charge of patients' safety issues, when prescribing to vulnerable, elderly dementia patients? How regularly are these reckless prescribing methods occurring?

These tragic events that happened to Judith occurred in the Isle of Man, but this was still an NHS qualified doctor; the UK NHS and

GMC has to take responsibility too. "Place of practice", should make no difference in the "standards of practice" and ethics. This evidence strongly highlights that Pharmacologists must play a role alongside Psychiatrists when a medication regime is classed as "polypharmacy"; even more so when "polypharmacy", is identified in a hospital environment. Patient safety must be a priority in Psychiatry too. Multiple qualifications and degrees are no substitute for a degree of common sense, where mere assumptions are made to the detriment of a patient.

I truly believe that the change in Judith's behaviour was a direct result of the plethora of medication that the Psychiatrist was prescribing her. We know that she had dementia, (most likely LBD), but I suspect that the long-term medication was in fact exasperating her condition too. Known common side-effects of Pregablin are, problems with memory or concentration; a totally inappropriate drug for a dementia patient then, and it is known to sometimes cause worsening symptoms in moods, depression, anxiety, agitation, hostility, aggressiveness and suicidal thoughts, amongst others. When mental health staff described Judith as "tortured", I would suggest this is exactly what she was; "tortured with medication".

The real, and most important question that needs to be asked, upon publication of this book is, "How many people actually know about Neuroleptic Malignant Syndrome?". There needs to be heightened awareness surrounding this illness, for the interests of public safety and to make fully informed decisions concerning dementia care.

Risperidone, I believe, should be banned for use in dementia patients. It has little benefit in my experience and The Banerjee Report, found that it is over-used in dementia patients, with very little benefit too. Since Judith's use of the drug, we saw only rapid progressive worsening of all symptoms. I suspect the benefits of Risperidone are hyped, and the success rates manipulated, for the sole purpose of increasing profits in the pharmaceutical industry. I seriously hope that my detailed account of Judith's death and the total lack of governance surrounding Risperidone and polypharmacy in dementia patients, along with the attempt at white-washing the safety issues by the Royal College of Psychiatrists, will put an end to the most concerning practice, when treating the elderly dementia population. As said, it is a problem that has been addressed previously by the UK Government and Professor Sube Banerjee, as detailed earlier, yet no implementation of the required governance has been put in place, to prevent this type of haphazard prescribing to dementia patients. Psychiatrists appear to be prescribing without any caution for the patient.

If your dog was ill, would you force an array of tablets down its throat and hope that one of them worked? If your dog then became even sicker, would you seriously know if it was the underlying illness that was getting worse, or if it was one of the tablets that caused further deteriorating health? That, to put it bluntly, is exactly what appears to be happening with dementia patients. The dangers of Risperidone in dementia patients are fully known.

We saw only a decline in Judith's behaviour and presentation during the periods of its use. No benefits were visible at all. Nobody in the Mental Health Unit could honestly say that Judith's behavioural symptoms improved during the periods of prescribing Risperidone. Unless, of course, total incapacitation is included in this. I have the MH records and saw no improvement in the catalogued entries by staff to support this. We knew that Judy had dementia, and would die of this disease in a few years, but the condition was exasperated cruelly, by the polypharmacy that she was subjected to.

Professor Ballard, a leading world-expert in dementia; Executive Dean of Medicine, University of Exeter (UK); a Professor of Old Age Psychiatry, disclosed that, "many people with Lewy Body dementia first come to hospital after being sectioned under the mental health act. The vast majority of Lewy Body dementia patients – 80 per cent – experience a very high frequency of distressing psychotic symptoms. Around a quarter of people diagnosed with LBD will have a reaction when given the wrong medication and may be misdiagnosed in up to 50 per cent of cases. Antipsychotics given to dementia sufferers to treat behavioural disturbances have been found to increase the risk of death fourfold, compared to one and a half times in people with Alzheimer's disease. They can also trigger a potentially fatal syndrome known as, "neuroleptic sensitivity reaction" – a very acute syndrome. Even if people do not die as a result of the syndrome, they may experience a steep decline in their condition, which they usually do not recover from". (Ref: www.independent.co.uk/news/health/lewy-body-dementia-prescription-antipsychotics-thousand-risk-injury-death-drugs-treatment-alzheimers-a7827431.html).

The "Time for Action" is now. Stop Risperidone usage in dementia patients. Their lives matter and Judith cannot be the only person to have been subjected to such appalling treatment. It is time for people to stand up for their rights; to say "No" to Risperidone, before it is too late.

The most important aspect of Judy's story is to highlight the condition of Neuroleptic Malignant Syndrome and help carers and family members to recognise the symptoms of this allegedly rare, but lethal illness, inflicted upon the patient by psychiatric medication. Literature details that fatality rates have in fact dropped drastically since early recognition of the onset of symptoms has increased. Yet, this book, highlights how easily it can be, and is overlooked. Early recognition of the syndrome and the halting of the antipsychotic drug risperidone is the single most important factor in aiding the patients' recovery. We, as healthy adults, or responsible carers or family members, should have the right to refuse ourselves or those we love, being subjected to Risperidone.

In my mother's case, the psychiatric statements that Judith was "highly unlikely", to have suffered from Neuroleptic Malignant Syndrome, was, following further research, incorrect at best.

Judith had delirium, as diagnosed by Psychiatry. This was never communicated by Mental Health to medics. No patient history was transferred from the unit. All patient history and details were needed to detect Neuroleptic Malignant Syndrome.

Judith's loss of mobility, consciousness and newly developed mutism was never passed to medics.

On Judith's first medical admission, no details of her fever, sweating and lack of breathing compliance was relayed from Mental Health. Her inability to drink fluid for nearly twenty four hours was never passed on either.

Swelling in Judith's neck noted by a nurse and a Health Care Assistant at Grianagh Court and in Judith's notes, was never communicated to medics.

Due to the full patient history and patient presentation information, not being given to the medical ward, the medics could not and did not identify delirium. Medics did not therefore stop delirium inducing medication.

Medics did declare that they had, "no idea", what was causing Judith's drowsiness, refusal to eat and her lack of balance. Babinski reflex signs in Judith were evident, suggesting central nervous system damage, which is associated with Neuroleptic Malignant Syndrome too.

Judith's refusal to eat, (anorexia), can be a result of suffering from Neuroleptic Malignant Syndrome; **lasting sequelae**, which Dr Mynors-Wallis and Dr Cope denied could happen in their professional report.

Judith developed a tremor, one day prior to her first hospital admission, and was prescribed Procyclidine. This was never relayed to medics. A tremor often is an early symptom of NMS also.

Most disturbing though, to counter the statement of "unlikely" NMS is:-

Judith was taking the antipsychotic drug, Risperidone, known to cause NMS.

She was taking Mirtazapine, known to bring on NMS.

She was taking donezepil (Aricept), known to induce NMS.

She was taking Sodium Valproate, known to precipitate NMS.

She was taking Furosemide – the ***only*** diuretic that increases mortality in patients taking Risperidone.

Yet Mental Health, Dr. Jagus and Dr Timothy Byrne both deemed it necessary to declare falsely, that Risperidone had not been taken, and had been stopped upon Judith's hospital admission. This despite the fact that Judith's level of polypharmacy had been noted as a "danger".

Therefore, in my opinion, the mental health services and the Isle of Man Hospital and Government ***employed*** Dr. Mynors-Wallis and Dr Cope to provide the professional report, (albeit marred), as a pinnacle to avoid any possible negligence allegations or corporate manslaughter allegations. They put Judith on the Liverpool Care Pathway, rather than treating her for undetected Neuroleptic Malignant Syndrome, and the remaining sequelae of such. (Interestingly, the Isle of Man has never changed the law like the UK, to allow Corporate Manslaughter to be a criminal charge).

No urinalysis had been carried out on Judith on her first admission to the medical ward, (or on her second admission), to prove the clinical diagnosis of a urine infection. Mental Health presumed Judith had a UTI on the basis that the urinalysis on 12 July 2012, (seven days earlier), was positive for E Choli, and antibiotics were prescribed at this point. The fact that no monitoring of the patient, (who was deemed to be "in danger of polypharmacy"), was ever undertaken; in addition to the Consultant Psychiatrist displaying no evidence of "caution" in his prescribing practices, which is detailed in the Patient Information Leaflets of many of the drugs that Judith was taking. Add to that, no patient history being provided by Mental Health to the Medical Ward and the Medical Ward being unable to access the patient's mental health records, it would appear glaringly obvious that Professor Sube Banerjee's statement is correct, "We need to make reductions in the use of these medications a clinical governance priority across the NHS". Dementia patients are dying from their failure to prioritise this. Therefore, each and every one of us, should have the right to refuse being treated with risperidone in the event that dementia takes hold. It is way too dangerous.

As sad as this book is, this is my desperate plea to stop this monstrous and reckless practice of torturing dementia patients further, with medication. As previously detailed, some of the drugs for dementia patients and depression associated with this, can cause cognitive impairment, aggression, mood swings, confusion, irritability and suicidal ideation.

Reform is seriously overdue and we must stop treating dementia patients and their families with such contempt and lack of governance. Failure to take steps towards clinical governance of these issues is tantamount to euthanasia, in my opinion. Judy cannot be the only patient to have endured such frivolous psychiatric prescribing practices. It MUST stop. Change is essential.

31

Questions to be Asked

Dementia is surely not just about medication is it?

When are we going to see recommendations of a high tryptophan diet to raise serotonin levels?

Research by John Hopkins Medicine into dementia in 2017 found low levels of serotonin in brain scans of dementia sufferers. The results suggest serotonin loss maybe a key player in cognitive decline, not just a side-effect of Alzheimer's disease. (www.sciencedaily.com/releases/2017/08/170814092943.htm).

Tryptophan increases serotonin levels. Serotonin levels lower as we age and low levels are linked to dementia. Therefore, a diet rich in tryptophans may benefit or delay dementia symptoms, especially cognitive decline and mood disturbances.

Foods rich in tryptophans are eggs, bananas, cheese, pineapples, tofu, nuts and seeds, salmon, turkey.

Although tryptophan high foods cannot raise serotonin levels alone, there is evidence that eating them with carbohydrates may boost levels. Eating tryptophans often with carbs such as rice, oatmeal and wholegrain bread should increase serotonin levels.

Other ways of raising serotonin levels are exercise, exposure to sun, eating a high-fibre diet to fuel healthy gut bacteria (PubMed Central-National Institute of Health).

There appear to be few studies on low serotonin levels in dementia that have been identified. Why is this not a field for further research?

Research has also shown that the risk for dementias is partially attributable to environmental factors – heavy metals, lead, cadmium and manganese are widespread and persistent in our environments.

Higher mercury concentrations were found in brain regions and blood of some patients with Alzheimer's Disease. Low levels of inorganic mercury were able to cause Alzheimer's Disease. (J Mutter et al. Fortst Neurol Psychiatry 2007 Sept).

B12 deficiency or B9 (called folate), deficiency anaemia occurs when a lack of B12 or folate causes the body to produce abnormally large red blood cells that cannot function properly.

Red blood cells carry oxygen around the body using a substance called haemoglobin.

Symptoms of vitamin B12 or folate deficiency include:

Extreme tiredness
A lack of energy
Pins and needles
A sore and red tongue
Muscle weakness
Disturbed vision

Psychological problems, which may include depression and confusion
Problems with memory, understanding and judgement

These conditions can often be diagnosed based on your symptoms and the results of a blood test.

It is important for vitamin B12 or folate deficiency anaemia to be diagnosed and treated as soon as possible. This is because although symptoms improve with treatment, some of the problems caused by the condition can be irreversible. (www.nhs.uk/conditions/vitamin-b12-or-folate-deficiency-anaemia/).

Humans used to obtain B12 from natural sources, like lakes, rivers and spring water. Although our water is now safer due to chlorination, it has eradicated any B12, so in-turn we look to animals who contain B12 and use their products as our source. Alternate vegan products are soy products and water lentils, (duckweed).

Vitamin B12 is exclusively made by microorganisms living in soil and water. It is not made by animals. It is obtained from the soil they digest with their food, as humans also did, from eating root vegetables with surface soil that were unwashed with chlorinated water, unlike modern times.

Vitamin B12 (Cobalamin) deficiency has been shown to be the most frequent associated physical disease in patients with dementia. The incidence of low vitamin B12 levels among dementia patients has been found to range between 29 per cent and 47 per cent. (The Journal of Neuropsychiatry. Norbert Goebels, M.D and Michael Soyka, M.D. (https://neuro.psychiatryonline.org/doi/full/10.1176/jnp.12.3.389).

Another dementia-like illness is idiopathic normal pressure hydrocephalus. The diagnosis is missed in 80 per cent of cases and is misdiagnosed as Alzheimer's disease or simply dementia. Yet idiopathic normal pressure hydrocephalus causing dementia is treatable, unlike many dementias.

So, what is idiopathic normal pressure hydrocephalus?

Normally the space between the brain and skull is filled with cerebrospinal fluid. It circulates and is gradually reabsorbed, but in normal pressure hydrocephalus the fluid is not reabsorbed. Therefore, when there is too much cerebrospinal fluid in and around the brain, it accumulates in the ventricles, and the brain is put under pressure, being pushed outwards, resulting in compression and damage of the brain.

Shunt surgery can rectify this condition, if diagnosed, normally by a neurologist, following a CT scan. (Dr. Vernon Coleman. When Dementia Can be Cured).

More recent studies have suggested a link between gum disease and dementia.

"The mouth is home to about 700 species of bacteria, including those that cause periodontal (gum), disease. A recent analysis led by NIA scientists suggests that bacteria that cause gum disease are also associated with the development of Alzheimer's disease and related dementias, especially vascular dementia. The results were published in the "Journal of Alzheimer's Disease".

Bacteria and the inflammatory molecules they make, can travel from infections in the mouth, through the blood stream to the brain". (Ref. www.nia.nih.gov/news/large-study-links-gum-disease-dementia).

Another substance gaining attention for treating Alzheimer's symptoms is Huperzine A, which is a substance purified from a plant called Chinese club moss. Huperzine A is used for Alzheimer's disease, memory, learning enhancement and age-related memory impairment.

In dementia, some research suggests that taking Huperzine A by mouth for up to 8 weeks may improve memory, mental function and behavior in people with conditions such as Alzheimer's or dementia. The long-term effects are not known.

With memory, research shows that taking Huperzine by mouth for 4 weeks improves the memory of older children and teenagers, complaining of memory problems.

(Ref. www.rxlist.com/huperzine_a/supplements.htm).

Always consult a doctor before taking any supplement or alternative medicine.

Again, as discussed earlier, a misdiagnosis of dementia can be a death sentence. As Professor Sube Banerjee's report detailed, "nearly 2,000 elderly patients are killed each year by unnecessary anti-psychotic medication".

Old age psychiatry should arrive at a diagnosis with neurologist input only.

Following a young woman dying in psychiatric care, the Senior Coroner, Inner London South, said there were inconsistencies when evidence was given to the Coroner's Court. Therefore, the Royal College of Psychiatrists' and the Royal College of Physicians' issued a joint statement on Neuroleptic Malignant Syndrome:-

Position Statement PS03/2014 December 2014

1. NMS is a rare and serious complication of antipsychotic therapy about which there is much uncertainty over definitions, cause, course and outcome. Nonetheless, all psychiatrists

practicing without immediate on-site supervision should be able to diagnose NMS.

2. NMS is best considered a medical emergency and is properly managed in an acute hospital. All medical staff in acute hospitals with responsibility for taking emergency referrals should know this and act accordingly. Acute clinicians should be prepared to accept cases of diagnosed NMS without reference to the current clinical state of the patient. Any debate over whether a patient should be transferred to the acute hospital should be about the issue of diagnosis only. Liaison psychiatry services within acute hospitals can manage the mental health needs of such patients, so these needs should never influence the decision to transfer. (www.rcpsych.ac.uk)

Clearly, antipsychotic medications cause NMS in young people too, let alone dementia patients.

Neuroleptic Malignant Syndrome is a very misunderstood condition, and I suspect still under-recognised and under-diagnosed too. Ever more incidents are being reported of the newer atypical antipsychotics, especially risperidone, being cited in cases of NMS.

The public have been misled by psychiatry, the pharmaceutical companies and the MHRA when we were led to believe that the newer atypical antipsychotics were safer, with fewer serious side-effects, especially NMS. There is increasing evidence that dehydration (this would include furosemide diuretic), whilst taking risperidone can induce NMS.

This begs the question, is this an appropriate and safe drug to prescribe to elderly dementia patients?

Remember, as previously detailed, it can take an average of eighteen months and three doctors to diagnose Lewy Body Dementia. Most of these patients are firstly mis-diagnosed as having Alzheimer's Dementia.

This book attempts to help demonstrate and identify the often lethal condition, both from a physical appearance angle, and from a medical criteria angle.

Due to the lack of clarity surrounding NMS, I hope to provide knowledge to both lay persons and medical professionals by telling Judith's story. Any heightened awareness of this condition will help future sufferers and their carers recognize symptoms, both family and institutionalized carers.

Author's Note

This account of Judith's experience has been told way too late. I apologise profusely for this. I found it difficult to recount, and aspects of this book I wished never to remember or relive. I know my daughter, Sophie, will shed many tears upon reading it, as I am sure, Judith's sister and extended family will too. My aim is not to cause distress in telling Judith's story, but to highlight the injustices that are happening when treating dementia patients, and to make anybody and everybody aware of the resounding effects that Psychiatry; the Pharmaceutical Industry and a lack of governance is having on dementia patients' latter years. We all die, but please afford us all some respect and dignity during the process.

At the time that this book was being published, Nigel had undergone treatment for Head and Neck cancer, at Clatterbridge Hospital. Following my previous hospital experiences, I can only say that my faith has been restored in our wonderful NHS system. Clatterbridge is full of staff who treat their patients with the utmost respect and positivity. Their professionalism, communication with, and friendliness towards their patients, is, in my limited experience, unprecedented. A big massive "thank you", to these amazing people and their upstanding ethics. They are a shining example of the cream of the best NHS system. Forever grateful. A big, big thank you to Doreen Wilkinson from the Isle of Man ENT unit and to Mr Lancaster at Aintree Hospital, who is an outstanding surgeon, oncologist, doctor and person. Forever grateful.

References and further reading

Caroff SN, Mann SC. Neuroleptic malignant syndrome. Med Clin North Am. 1993;77:185 – 202. [PubMed]

Caroff SN, Mann SC, Campbell EC. Atypical antipsychotics and neuroleptic malignant syndrome. Psychiatr Ann. 2000;30:314 – 21.

Caroff SN. Neuroleptic malignant syndrome [Still a risk but which patient may be in danger?] Curr Psychiatr. 2003;12:36 – 42.

Davis JM, Caroff SN, Mann SC. Treatment of neuroleptic malignant syndrome. Psychiatr Ann. 2000;30:325 – 31.

Fink M. Neuroleptic malignant syndrome and catatonia: one entity or two? Biol Psychiatry. 1996;39:1 – 4. [PubMed]

Levenson JL. Neuroleptic malignant syndrome. Am J Psychiatry. 1985;142:1137 – 45. [PubMed]

Shalev A, Hermesh H, Munitz H. Mortality from neuroleptic malignant syndrome. J Clin Psychiatry 1989; 50:18.

Velamoor VR. Neuroleptic malignant syndrome. Recognition, prevention and management. Drug Saf 1998; 19:73.

Margetić B, Aukst-Margetić B. Neuroleptic malignant syndrome and its controversies. Pharmacoepidemiol Drug Saf 2010; 19:429.

Keck PE Jr, Pope HG Jr, Cohen BM, et al. Risk factors for neuroleptic malignant syndrome. A case-control study. Arch Gen Psychiatry 1989; 46:914.

Chandran GJ, Mikler JR, Keegan DL. Neuroleptic malignant syndrome: case report and discussion. CMAJ 2003; 169:439.

Strawn JR, Keck PE Jr, Caroff SN. Neuroleptic malignant syndrome. Am J Psychiatry 2007; 164:870.

Seitz DP, Gill SS. Neuroleptic malignant syndrome complicating antipsychotic treatment of delirium or agitation in medical and surgical patients: case reports and a review of the literature. Psychosomatics 2009; 50:8.

Pope HG Jr, Aizley HG, Keck PE Jr, McElroy SL. Neuroleptic malignant syndrome: long-term follow-up of 20 cases. J Clin Psychiatry 1991; 52:208.

Hermesh H, Aizenberg D, Weizman A, et al. Risk for definite neuroleptic malignant syndrome. A prospective study in 223 consecutive in-patients. Br J Psychiatry 1992; 161:254.

Berardi D, Amore M, Keck PE Jr, et al. Clinical and pharmacologic risk factors for neuroleptic malignant syndrome: a case-control study. Biol Psychiatry 1998; 44:748.

Koch M, Chandragiri S, Rizvi S, et al. Catatonic signs in neuroleptic malignant syndrome. Compr Psychiatry 2000; 41:73.

Adnet P, Lestavel P, Krivosic-Horber R. Neuroleptic malignant syndrome. Br J Anaesth 2000; 85:129.

Lee JW. Serum iron in catatonia and neuroleptic malignant syndrome. Biol Psychiatry 1998; 44:499.

Gurrera RJ, Caroff SN, Cohen A, et al. An international consensus study of neuroleptic malignant syndrome diagnostic criteria using the Delphi method. J Clin Psychiatry 2011; 72:1222.

Tural U, Onder E. Clinical and pharmacologic risk factors for neuroleptic malignant syndrome and their association with death. Psychiatry Clin Neurosci 2010; 64:79.

Trollor JN, Sachdev PS. Electroconvulsive treatment of neuroleptic malignant syndrome: a review and report of cases. Aust N Z J Psychiatry 1999; 33:650.

Caroff SN, Mann SC, Keck PE Jr, Francis A. Residual catatonic state following neuroleptic malignant syndrome. J Clin Psychopharmacol 2000; 20:257.

Nakamura M, Yasunaga H, Miyata H, et al. Mortality of neuroleptic malignant syndrome induced by typical and atypical antipsychotic drugs: a propensity-matched analysis from the Japanese Diagnosis Procedure Combination database. J Clin Psychiatry 2012; 73:427. www.patient.co.uk/doctor/neuroleptic-malignant-syndrome.

Davis JM, Janicak PG, Sakkas P, Gilmore C, Wang Z. Electroconvulsive therapy in the treatment of the neuroleptic malignantsyndrome. Convuls Ther 1991;7:111 – 120.

Ananth J, Parameswaran S, Gunatilake S, Burgoyne K, Sidhom T. Neuroleptic malignant syndrome and atypical antipsychotic drugs. J Clin Psychiatry 2004;65:464 – 70.

Made in the USA
Monee, IL
04 November 2026

67384624R00167